LESSONS FROM A GENTLE LIFE

Early Praise for *Lessons from a Gentle Life*

"*Lessons from a Gentle Life* is a poignant sharing of hard-earned wisdom gained on many levels. Lessons of living more deeply after the death of your precious child co-exist with lessons of how we can be more fully human in this world and how we can grow to understand our own failings and strengths through profound loss. I felt every word in my cells and have lived so many moments of Janis's path. *Lessons from a Gentle Life* is a beautiful testament to Cariana's life and the immense difference a short, young life so wisely lived can make in this world."

> ~Shari O'Loughlin, Executive Director, Children's Grief Center of NM; Bereaved Mom; Author of *Life from the Ashes; Finding Signs of Hope After Loss*

"Hope glows from the pages of this intimate narrative from a mother who has walked the pathway that parents fear most of all. With grace, sensitivity, and humor, Janis Gonzales shares tender insights about the heights and depths of love, and the realities of grief. Her story reminds us that life calls each of us to face the challenges of transformation, and her hard-won perspective gifts us with wisdom about how to make that journey: what to surrender along the way, and just as importantly, what to safeguard forever in the beating chambers of our hearts."

> ~Kathryn Lynard, author of *Gifts: Mothers Reflect on How Children with Down Syndrome Enrich Their Lives*

"Weaving together her wisdom for both mothering and medicine, Dr. Gonzales creates a beautiful tapestry of loss, love and hope. She takes us to that 'razor's edge between joy and sorrow' using threads from her personal heartache and tender intuition, as well as literature and science. No matter what your life circumstances might be, Dr. Gonzales's writing invites reflection. By the end of the book, I felt the warm weight and deep spirit of her daughter, as if she were in my own arms calling me to life."
~Rev. Linda C. Loving, Presbyterian Pastor and author of *A New Song to Sing: Breast Cancer as Journey of Spirit*

"Staying true to Cariana's legacy, with artistic skill, Janis weaves in and out of a beautiful love story between her and her precious daughter. As she draws us into her unimaginable heartache, she brings hope and comfort to anyone who has experienced loss. I highly recommend this gift of healing."
~Cathy Chavez, R.N., oncology nurse and author of *Hold Every Moment Sacred*

"Beautiful and inspiring, the author generously shares her story in a way that allows readers to witness her pain and growth and thereby apply her lessons to our own lives. With a subtle and gentle humor, cleverly weaving her own story in with data and reflections on the world of medicine, the author offers a unique perspective on life, death and grief. In a time when compassion and understanding is so needed in the world, Dr. Gonzales delivers with this book."
~Giovanna Rossi, MSc
President, Collective Action Strategies, LLC
Leadership Consultant and Transformation Coach

LESSONS FROM A GENTLE LIFE

Reflections on Love, Loss and Healing

JANIS GONZALES, MD

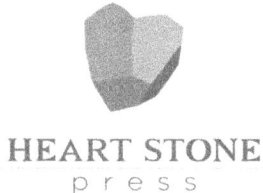

HEART STONE
press

All rights reserved.

Except for use in a review, no part of this book may be reproduced, in whole or in part, including text, photographs, illustrations, and artwork, in any form or by any means, electronic or mechanical, including photocopying, recording, or any information storage and retrieval system except by expressed written permission from the publisher.

Copyright © 2019 Janis Gonzales, MD

Published by
HeartStonePress
223 N Guadalupe #104
Santa Fe NM 87501
www.HeartStonePress.com

Cover: Leslie Waltzer, Crowfoot Design
Cover photo: David Gonzales, MD

Printed and bound in USA

Library of Congress Control Number: 2019905389

ISBN
978-1-7331427-0-0 (paperback)
978-1-7331427-1-7 (ebook/mobi)
978-1-7331427-2-4 (ebook/epub)

Disclaimer: The information in this book is not intended to diagnose, treat, cure, or prevent any disease and is not intended as a substitute for the medical advice of physicians or professional care. The reader should consult a physician in matters relating to his/her or a family member's health and particularly with respect to any symptoms that may require diagnosis or medical attention.

For Cariana, who taught me how to love, and Placido and Liesl, who continue to help me deepen that love every day.

CONTENTS

Introduction- 11

Part One

Lightning Strikes- 15

The Blessings of an Imperfect Life- 33

Practicing Medicine- 47

To Hope or Not to Hope- 55

Part Two

A Grief Observed- 65

Part Three

Growing Pains- 77

Signs of Life- 85

Unexpected Gifts- 99

Alchemy- 107

Epilogue- 113

Acknowledgments- 115

About the Author- 117

Introduction

It often happens in life that we plan to do one thing and end up doing another. I set out to write a book about my daughter, Cariana, the relationship we shared together, and how that relationship changed me; about modern medicine, and doctoring, and how learning to care for patients in no way teaches you how to heal yourself or your child. The book you are holding in your hand does cover those things; but in the ten years between the first and second drafts, a larger theme of resiliency and transformation has become interwoven through it all.

This book, at its core, is about acceptance. Accepting who we are, with all our faults, insecurities and imperfections. Accepting what life gives us, even if it doesn't fit with the life we had planned. Accepting others by learning to value each person we meet without pre-judging their abilities. Accepting that no matter how hard we try, we will never be able to control everything that happens to us in life, and that the only thing we really can control is the lesson we choose to take from our experiences. Accepting that even though loving deeply opens us up to deep sorrow, it also opens us to living fully and authentically.

The first draft of this book was started during Cariana's illness, scribbled in a spiral notebook I kept with me during the long hours at the hospital. In our quiet room, while she slept, I would jot down notes about our experiences. That notebook turned into a manuscript in the months after Cariana's death when all I could do was write, and cry, and write some more. Stephen King said it best: "Writing is not life, but I think that sometimes it can be a way back to life." Writing was the one thing that got me out of bed every day. It was a way to preserve an experience that was both painful and precious.

With the help of an agent, I sent that manuscript to a few publishers without success. Eventually I turned my attention to other things: mothering two still-small children, dealing with the legalities of divorce, and focusing on the full-time job my new status as a single parent required. Ten years somehow went by before I took the manuscript out again. But over those ten years I had amassed a pile of notes and random thoughts, some printed from emails and my iPhone notepad, some scribbled on church bulletins and fast food napkins. Those notes added immeasurably to the finished product, making it a compilation of two very different emotional states: the bitter, raw grief of a mother whose child has just died in her arms and the hard-won peace and serenity that only time and tears can bring.

Cariana was born on August 29, two weeks before 9/11. In many ways, during the time period covered in this book, our country has collectively been going through a post-traumatic stress response right along with me. I don't have a silver bullet that will cure everything we have gone through, and everything we continue to go through, but I've heard it said that if the book you want to read doesn't exist, you must write it, and that's what I did. It is the book I needed to read fourteen years ago but was unable to find.

Part One

Dreadful is the mysterious power of Fate;
there is no escape from it by wealth or war,
by walled city, or dark, sea-beaten ships.

-Sophocles
Antigone

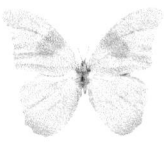

~Lightning Strikes~

In the early morning light, the spots were barely visible. Cariana was playing happily on the floor, putting plastic gold coins into a slit in a wooden box, when I noticed the red pinpoint dots faintly scattered on the soft skin just above her pink flowered socks. Pressing on the rash I observed, incredulously, that it didn't blanch, which meant that the spots were actually petechiae, tiny hemorrhages in the skin. In my eight years as a pediatrician I had seen several children with that kind of rash, but although I had studied the possible causes, I had never quite gotten over the sense of dread that comes with each encounter.

My mind flipped through options like the flickering scenes of a movie reel, and I chose denial, at least for the moment. If I had examined a child in my office with a rash like that, I would have told the parents to go directly to the lab to obtain a platelet count. But I wasn't ready to start down that road. We continued our day as planned – reading, playing, running errands, and doing everything I could think of to distract myself from what was happening to Cariana.

I managed to get through most of the day without directly looking at her, but by 4:00 in the afternoon I could no longer avoid seeing the obvious: the rash was spreading. Picking her up carefully, I buckled her into her car seat and headed over to the office to see my partner, who was finishing up with his last few patients of the day.

Larry and I had been working together for eight years. I had decreased my work schedule a little bit more with each pregnancy, so that now, with three children, I seemed to spend more time in the office as a mother than I did as a pediatrician. Larry had been great about accepting all my childbearing decisions, despite the fact that I had brought every baby to him in turn, convinced that each one had some kind of bizarre neurological or developmental disorder. When our son Placido was nine months old, Dave and I were sure his facial contortions were atypical seizures, and even insisted that Larry watch the videotape we had made as evidence. That video got us our first specialty referral to a pediatric neurologist in Albuquerque who shrugged and said he had no idea what the "episodes" were. Luckily, they never recurred.

Sixteen months later Liesl was born, and one of the first things I noticed, after she crawled up onto my chest in search of milk, was a classic, hypo-pigmented "ash leaf spot" on her back. This prompted Dave and I to scrutinize her closely for months, each of us secretly convinced that she was destined to develop tuberous sclerosis. This time, although we were quick to point out the spot to Larry at every check-up, we held off on the dermatology referral he gave us and decided to just keep on eye on Liesl's development – which, of course, turned out to be completely normal.

Now, it was Cariana's turn, and I was hoping against hope that my suspicions would be proven false again.

"I'm probably just overreacting," I told him, trying to sound as if I thought that was a genuine possibility.

Larry looked Cariana over and was silent for a moment. Denial was looking really good to him, too.

Sitting in the orange vinyl chairs of the familiar, cozy waiting room, my mind flashed back to the day Cariana was born, almost two years ago. Although we violated the speed limit as much as we dared and ran every red light we encountered on the way to the hospital, we got there just in time for the delivery. My plans for an epidural went out the window as the nurses rushed to get me into a room. In fifteen minutes, Cariana was born. Only in retrospect did I realize the room was strangely silent.

The obstetrician left quickly, and I cradled Cariana in my arms. She looked at me with luminous, slanted eyes that twinkled, as if she had a secret she wasn't quite ready to share with me. In my blissful, hormone-saturated state, I didn't notice anything wrong as I breastfed Cariana and she wrapped her tiny hand around my finger. The experienced delivery room nurse immediately suspected that this was a baby with Down syndrome, but protocol demanded that she wait for the pediatrician to do his exam. She was very kind, but I thought it slightly odd that she kept walking in and out of the room, glancing at me tentatively out of the corner of her eye and repeatedly asking me if I was *sure* everything was ok.

A couple of hours later, Larry came in on his morning rounds to examine Cariana. I watched him impatiently, wondering why in the world he was spending so much time on a newborn physical. Finally, he turned and said, "The nurse thought there was something wrong, but I think she's fine." And I was so happy to have her back in my arms, 95 percent of me actually believed him.

Now, almost two years later, I could laugh at the thought that we were ever sad about Cariana having Down syndrome. It was just a part of who she was, and we loved everything about her: her beautiful, ever-present smile; her big, sparkling brown eyes that always seem amused; her small white teeth that had erupted in erratic order; her sweet little voice; and her dolphin laugh (which was almost identical to Liesl's).

Everything, that is, except for those darn spots that were covering her arms and legs. When I left the office with Cariana, Larry said he would get us an appointment with a dermatologist for the following morning – his way of passing the buck so he wouldn't have to be the bearer of the bad news. In the morning, however, Larry had a change of heart. Just as we were packing up to leave for the appointment, he called me on my cell phone to ask me to take Cariana to the lab for a stat CBC.

The lab was sterile and white except for one small "children's room" that was decorated with colorful drawings of rainbows and animal mobiles that hung from the ceiling. It smelled faintly of rubbing alcohol mixed with diaper cream. The lab tech had to call for help, which didn't surprise me since I knew from experience that drawing blood on a not-quite-two-year-old girl is a bit like trying to suck juice from an apple with a cocktail straw.

By the time Cariana and I left the lab we were both drenched with sweat, but I picked up Dave and we headed over to the dermatologist's office to keep our appointment. We arrived a few minutes early, and as we waited in the car, Cariana fell asleep in my arms, totally oblivious to the turmoil the rest of us were feeling. The seconds ticked by on my five-dollar Target wristwatch as I played with the silver band nervously.

Finally, just as we got out of the car and started to approach the office door, we saw Larry walking towards us, holding the test results in his hand.

He had the stricken look of a flight attendant announcing that the plane you are on has just been hijacked, and instead of going to Boston you're going to be taking a little detour to Peru.

Cariana's blood cell counts were all abnormally low, especially the platelets. Instead of going into the office to see the dermatologist, we drove home to make an appointment with the pediatric oncologist, the one specialist every parent lives in fear of ever having to meet.

On the drive from Santa Fe to the University of New Mexico oncology clinic in Albuquerque, Dave and I sat stiffly, conversation lapsing into long silences. Cariana fussed occasionally in her car seat, just to make sure we were still aware of her presence. We knew just where to go – the parking garage across the street, the red bridge we needed to walk across to get to the pediatric clinic – because we had done it all before, two years earlier, when we came to consult with the geneticist.

The waiting room in the Pediatric Specialty Clinic was full, and the wait was going to be long. I wasn't sure if it was because Dave and I were both physicians or because they were so worried about Cariana's condition, but despite having a full schedule, they were squeezing us in for the procedure that would tell us what was going on in Cariana's bone marrow.

The clinic was bustling, and the first thing I noticed was that the other parents in the waiting room weren't crying. Instead of looking sad, the other mothers were laughing, knitting and gossiping like Mrs. Kravitz on *Bewitched*. It was incredible. "Don't they understand what's happening?" I wondered.

I had that sinking feeling you get in your stomach when you know you've been suckered into doing something you don't want to do and there is no way out. Then it hit me out of the blue, what I later found out was an extremely common reaction among parents in our situation: the simple, overwhelming urge to pick my child up and get away from this place, these people, as fast as I could.

I had completely lost my sense of what comprised "normal" behavior. It honestly didn't seem to me that the idea of running far away with my sick child was irrational. At that moment I would probably have said that it sounded perfectly reasonable to climb Mt. Everest wearing only a loincloth or style my hair with a roto-tiller. I would have entered the Iditarod if I thought it would get us out of there.

All the children in the waiting room were bald, the one unmistakable sign of cancer. As I watched them I thought back to the children I had cared for as a pediatric resident. I remembered my fear that I would never know enough, never be good enough. I didn't want to hurt anybody. I didn't want to make any mistakes.

As a resident it had been painful to see children suffer. It was even harder to realize that not all of their suffering was attributable to their illness. We inflicted much of it ourselves as part of their treatment. The drugs we gave them sometimes made them sicker, at least temporarily; and the procedures, though necessary, caused them pain and filled their eyes with fear. I had chosen pediatrics for its optimism, and I hadn't expected the surprising sadness that stayed with me after I went home at night.

The pediatric oncologists, on the other hand, showed no outward signs of sadness. Everyone we met that day was cheerful, almost ebullient. We were a little taken aback, however, when a man with short hair walked into the room where we were waiting with Cariana. Wearing a tight black T-shirt, a colorful biker tattoo on his arm, and a birthday crown on his head, he announced brightly that he was going to be her doctor. That was our introduction to Dr M, Cariana's oncologist, who happened to be celebrating his 50th birthday.

Once we got over the initial shock of his appearance, we found Dr. M to be optimistic, friendly and deeply caring. Looking back on it now, I think it's possible the other doctors in the clinic may have assigned him to our case on purpose as a kind of birthday joke. Of course, no one ever said as much. But doctors are notorious for being terrible patients, and I'm pretty sure no one in the clinic that day was excited about taking on the care of a little girl who had two physicians for parents.

It took several tries with the bone marrow needle to get enough marrow for the aspirate and the biopsy. The IV dripped interminably. Cariana tolerated everything well, sleeping peacefully (under sedation) throughout the entire procedure. Unfortunately for me, I wasn't offered the same option. I could have used some sedation myself – or, at the very least, a frozen and unnaturally blue concoction served in a hollowed-out pineapple with a tiny umbrella stuck in it.

We were taken down the hall to the clinic recovery area, where several other (mostly hairless) children of various ages were sitting around, casually chatting while getting their doses of chemotherapy and munching on popcorn and turkey sandwiches. The movie "Aladdin" was playing on a big screen TV in the corner. A nurse came to check Cariana's vital signs. Coming out of the propofol haze, she reacted crazily, swinging her arms, pushing me away, and crying. I struggled with her, trying to hold her tightly so she wouldn't fall off the bed.

For years after finishing college I had suffered from a recurring nightmare in which I showed up for a final exam, only to realize with dread that I had forgotten all about the class and hadn't attended it all semester. Recently I had been having a new dream, one in which I unexpectedly found myself at the starting line of a marathon that I hadn't trained for, and everyone was expecting me to win.

All I kept thinking was that I wanted to go home – as if just getting back there would magically end the nightmare and everything would be normal again. I didn't comprehend yet just how drastically all our lives were about to change.

We had to wait five agonizing days for the pathologists to decide exactly what was wrong with Cariana's bone marrow. As it turned out, her bone marrow was so unusual that they couldn't have just one pathologist look at it – they had to get every pathologist in the group to examine it under the microscope and even confer with experts at other centers. Frustrated with the glacial movement of the pathology department, I phoned the on-call pediatric oncologist Thursday, Friday, Saturday and Sunday asking for results. Each time, the oncologists patiently explained to me that although they were there working on the weekend, the pathologists were not.

Physicians who have not been patients themselves often underestimate the stress of waiting for results. We get used to the idea that accurate test results take time, and we think that waiting several days or even a week for test results is routine; while at home, our patients are anxiously pacing up and down, staring at the phone and willing it to ring, unable to concentrate on anything else.

As two physicians, you might assume that Dave and I would have been prepared to wait several days for the bone marrow results, but you would be wrong. When your own child is the one undergoing the tests, having to wait even one day for results is far too long. We were trapped in a Dickensian nightmare, dreading the words that would be spoken by the impending Spirits but wanting to get it all over with at the same time.

I was angry, with no outlet for my anger, and my frustration echoed Placi's own outbursts. He had been quiet and shy as a toddler, and his first couple of years were most memorable for his tendency to creep out of his bed and fall asleep in the hallway, blankie by his side, stretched out prone on the carpet like a human speed bump. Placi at age six was extremely bright and curious about everything, constantly asking questions and already reading well above his grade level. But for several months now, despite his predominantly sweet and helpful nature, I had been worried about his temper tantrums, which seemed to come out of nowhere.

Liesl, always the peacemaker, came into the kitchen after Placi had been sent to his room.

"It's ok, Mama," she told me seriously. "Placi will break your heart, and I will fix it."

When the phone rang, I jumped. My heart pounded. It was Mom calling, hopeful that maybe we had received some results and just forgotten to tell her.

"Maybe the sprinklers went off in the pathology lab and they're still drying everything out," I hypothesized.

"I'm sure they'll call soon," Mom said, ignoring my sarcasm.

As I hung up the phone, I swallowed hard, relieved that, at least for today, Placi was not asking for explanations of things I knew I could not explain.

Two days later the pathologists finally came to a consensus on the diagnosis: high-grade myelodysplastic syndrome, also known as MDS. MDS in children is rare and poorly understood. I racked my brain to try to recall hearing about it somewhere in medical school or residency and silently berated myself for not memorizing the Pediatric Oncology textbook.

MDS is not leukemia, they told us, but it can be a precursor to it in about 20% of cases. In the typical pediatric population, acute lymphocytic leukemia (ALL) is much more common than acute myelogenous leukemia (AML) – about a 4:1 ratio throughout most of childhood. But in children with Down syndrome, the ratio is approximately 1:1. This means that not only are children with Down syndrome more likely to develop leukemia, but they are also significantly more likely to develop the AML type of leukemia.

My ears took in this information from the oncologists, but my mind was having difficulty processing it.

"At least it isn't leukemia," I thought to myself.

But what exactly was it? And how bad could it be if Cariana didn't have any symptoms?

Placi heard us talking on the phone and asked me, "Mommy, what is happening in Cariana's bones?"

This seemed to me an unanswerable question, like asking who created Stonehenge or what really caused the crop circles. Perhaps there was some PBS show we could watch that would clarify it.

"It's hard to explain, buddy" was all I could say.

Cariana's bone marrow showed the cytopenias and blasts expected in MDS, but it also demonstrated multiple, atypical chromosomal abnormalities. This, according to her pathology report, indicated "a high degree of chromosome instability" and was felt be a signal of a rapidly evolving process, meaning that there was the potential for her to get worse quickly.

The protocol recommended for Cariana would involve six cycles of chemotherapy, ranging in length from four days to two weeks per cycle. Each round would be scheduled approximately one month apart, although the actual timing would depend on how fast her bone marrow recovered in between, as measured by her blood cell counts. The oncologists told us that the chemotherapy would temporarily wipe out the normal blood cells being produced in Cariana's bone marrow, and that afterwards, her cell counts would remain low for several days to weeks, leaving her susceptible to severe infections and vulnerable to needing frequent transfusions.

When the oncologist called us with the final report saying that Cariana had myelodysplastic syndrome, my first question to him was "Are they sure?" I was actually hoping for uncertainty. There was no room anymore for wishful thinking, no chance to deny the reality of the diagnosis and what it meant. We had the answer. We couldn't pretend Cariana was still ok.

Cariana had already beaten the odds at birth. Almost fifty percent of babies with Down syndrome have some kind of congenital heart defect; many others have intestinal problems, thyroid disease, cataracts, or any of a number of other ailments. It's not uncommon for children with Down syndrome to need surgery or be hospitalized frequently, but aside from a couple of ear infections Cariana had been completely healthy.

Of course, that was all before - on the "Before" side of the "Before and After" mark that had suddenly and indelibly been drawn through the timeline of my life. That was before, when we were like so many other people, doing our chores and going to our jobs and taking care of our beautiful, healthy children. That was before I understood how one tiny thing could ruin everything, like a hairline crack in a crystal glass, or a tiny red spot on a child's leg just above her ruffled sock; how the world could be irreversibly changed by a test result; how one breath could bring down the whole house of cards.

I stared at Cariana dazedly, still amazed to think how much

I loved her and how, incredibly, she seemed to love me back with equal adoration. I had felt this way with every baby: awed by my capacity to love another person more than I ever thought possible. Over and over, in the midst of doing some insignificant thing like folding her laundry, or packing her diaper bag, or putting her soft pink slippers on her tiny feet, the realization would hit me like a wave, and I would suddenly feel the strength of our connection and the depth of our love.

It was just so hard to believe. She looked so happy and she didn't appear to have any discomfort whatsoever. On the outside she was smiling, learning, growing, developing. But inside her very bones, her body was failing.

I spent hours on the Internet, searching for any available treatment options. I knew that The Answer to this new problem had to exist out there somewhere and that I could find it if I just worked hard enough and searched long enough. I joined listservs, pulled up every article on pediatric MDS written in the past decade, and wrote to pediatric leukemia specialists all over the country. Amazingly, every one of them emailed me back, a testament to the generosity and extraordinary kindness of the people who choose to work in the field of pediatric oncology.

When Cariana was diagnosed her doctors estimated the odds of a cure to be 75%. To most people that would sound pretty good, but I knew better: that number meant nothing. My child was born with Down syndrome, and the odds of that were one in 400. Then she developed leukemia, and the odds of that were 1 in 150. A husband and wife in Belmont, California each bought winning lottery tickets the same day, an outcome calculated at 1 in 23 trillion. The odds of something happening were completely meaningless once it had happened to you.

What was next? Falling down a manhole? Disappearing through a rift in the space-time continuum? I felt as if anything could happen, as if I was a magnet for all the possible illnesses and tragedies that could occur in life. In ancient Greek mythology, when someone died suddenly, they were said to have been struck by Apollo's arrow. I could almost hear Apollo sneaking around, snickering in the shadows.

Before Cariana could get started on the chemo, she had to have a central line put in. The one we chose was called a Broviac and is basically like a large IV where the chemo would enter her body, which would hopefully preserve her tiny peripheral veins. But watching a Broviac being inserted in medical school in no way prepares you for the reality of seeing your own child being given chemotherapy.

The universe felt dangerous and unpredictable. Taking care of children was my job—both as a mother and a pediatrician. It was shattering to think that I couldn't protect her.

After the surgery, Cariana's eyes were still puffy from the extra fluids they had given her. Dressed in a flowered hospital gown, she shivered a little. I wrapped my arms around her tightly. A smiling nurse, who seemed suspiciously cheery, hung the orange chemo bag on Cariana's IV pole. It was labeled "DANGER: TOXIC WASTE." Suddenly it occurred to me that I had spent the past two years feeding my daughter organic baby food and nurturing her with my own milk, and now I was expected to just stand back and allow these smiling strangers to drip poison into her veins.

During our second visit to the oncology clinic they had given us a copy of the entire treatment protocol, which listed all the possible side effects of the chemotherapy medications. They included "diarrhea, rash, nausea, vomiting, back or neck pain, headache, confusion, tiredness, seizures, slurred speech, partial paralysis, low blood counts, mouth sores, hair loss, eye irritation, fever, bone pain, poor brain function, inflammation of the lungs, difficulty breathing, stiff neck, damage to brain tissue, and unsteady gait."

In Stephen Sondheim's Into the Woods, the witch sings: "Children can only grow from something you love to something you lose." The possibility of loss hovered over Cariana's crib like the vultures over the Towers of Silence. "This is too hard," I wanted to scream. "I can't stay here." The thought of doing this for the next 6 months seemed unimaginable. Teresa, the mother of a beautiful young girl with AML, came to introduce herself and said gently, "The beginning is the worst." I just stared at her implacably, not knowing how to answer.

People kept coming by, bearing gifts – homemade blankets, stuffed animals, toys. The social worker, Gina, helpfully delivered a 5-inch thick notebook in which to keep the protocol "roadmap", emergency phone numbers, hospital information, and all of Cariana's test results. My anxiety was palpable; it wrapped around me like a quilt as I hunkered down in the rocking chair, cuddling Cariana, barely speaking to anyone.

I wasn't sure I wanted to meet any more parents whose children had AML or MDS. According to the statistics Dr. M had given us, one out of every four of those children would not survive long-term. I had met more than four children with leukemia already. I wondered which ones weren't going to make it, and if there was any way to tell.

It was a question that had haunted me since medical school: how do we explain the fact that two people with the same disease, who received exactly the same treatment, could have such different outcomes? It wasn't even Darwinian—the strongest didn't necessarily survive. I had seen some kids who looked so fragile, like they were close to death, and they still pulled through. Others looked so hale and hearty you could hardly believe they were ill, and they turned out to be the sickest of all. It wasn't survival of the fittest; it was survival of the random and the lucky.

Knowing there was a possibility of losing her, I looked at each day with Cariana as a precious gift. But I couldn't help wondering how I could pack a lifetime of hugs and kisses into just a few months. I desperately wished I could save her hugs the way we used to save green stamps, pasting them into books so I could retrieve them when I needed to feel her little arms around me in the future.

Cariana had finished almost 48 hours of chemo and she hadn't even thrown up, which I took to be a good sign that she would tolerate the treatment protocol without too many side effects. She was doing so well that we were already planning to bring her home immediately after the 96-hour infusion was completed.

The oncologist on the ward that week gave her excellent medical care. He was very thorough and a stickler for detail, always making sure that we were following the protocol to the letter, which I really appreciated. I didn't think he liked me, however. I got the feeling he thought I was being a tad unrealistic. Several times, he came into the room and told me not to expect too much.

"I have 14 years of experience," he warned me repeatedly, "and most of the children need to stay at least an extra day or two."

Cariana stopped breastfeeding for a second and grinned up at him as if telling him not to worry so much. When she finished the milk, she ate an entire plate of spaghetti. Sitting in her bed, she turned the pages of her Runaway Bunny book and chattered away. As she finished the book she tossed it out of the crib and laughed. She was entertaining herself so well that I was thinking of leaving the room for a minute, when I happened to glance over and saw something thin and white lying there on the bed next to her.

The Broviac was out.

That was the last straw. All the emotions that had been smoldering inside me suddenly exploded. I was angry at everyone and everything. It is said that having a child with a disability is the best assertiveness-training course there is. Having a child with a disability anda life-threatening illness, I felt like I hadn't just taken a training course in assertiveness, I had gotten a Ph.D.

My precious child had already had her tender skin scarred with multiple punctures for IV's and blood draws over the past few weeks. Now we were right back where we started, having to hold her down and stab her with needles again, not to mention a second surgery when she had barely recovered from the first.

I pushed the call button as forcefully as humanly possible, and soon various pediatric and surgical residents came traipsing in to stare at Cariana as if she was a rare species of tropical fish. The residents were followed by two nurses, an X-ray technician, the oncologist, the surgeon, and several visitors from down the hall who poked their heads in to see what the commotion was all about. It was St. Elsewhere: the Lost Episode. The fourth time someone asked, "Did she pull her line out?" I completely lost it.

"She did NOT pull on it! IT JUST FELL OUT!!!!"

I knew everyone thought I was rude, but I didn't care. I was holding myself together with Scotch tape.

Over the next few months we made so many trips to the hospital the staff began to feel like a second family. I liked hearing their muffled voices out at the nurses' station, but it was hard not to wish I could be out there with them. After all, that had been my usual place for years whenever I was in a hospital – sitting behind the desk, checking lab results, writing orders.

Even though I loved being with Cariana, I wasn't used to being stuck in a cramped room for hours on end. I was used to being the one writing the orders. Now I kept wondering what orders were secretly being written without my knowledge. It was junior high all over again. They were the popular kids whispering together, and I was the one standing by my locker knowing I wouldn't be invited to the party they were planning.

Given my earlier behavior, I figured I was lucky if the oncologists didn't duck into the video closet or dive out the nearest window when they saw me coming. I stayed with Cariana, bivouacked in that little room with my stash of snacks and magazines. The nurses were friendly and courteous, but I was sure they were secretly whispering behind my back, wondering where I went to medical school and sighing loudly over the fact that I had obviously not applied myself.

I didn't even understand how to care for the Broviac. Maybe it was the thick fog of sleep deprivation, but it seemed incredibly complicated. This topic had never been addressed in any of my med school courses or in the baby books littering my shelves at home. Ironically, I felt completely unprepared to go home and care for a sick child. No one had given me a copy of What to Expect During Your Child's First Year with Cancer, with chapters like "101 Ways to get your Son to Take His Medicine" and "Your Daughter's Central Line: Friend or Foe?"

In some ways, though, I didn't really mind staying in the hospital all that much. Cariana and I loved each other so much, it didn't really matter to us where we were as long as we were together, talking and smiling and absorbing each other's love. We were as closely connected as it is possible for two people to be, a blessing I knew I did not deserve. But love, it turns out, isn't given to the deserving. It's serendipity and grace. It doesn't come because of who we are, but in spite of it.

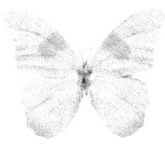

~The Blessings of an Imperfect Life~

A friend of mine used to try to decide the future of his romantic relationships by statistical analysis of what he liked and disliked about each person, complete with colorful graphs and charts listing things like what he had in common with each one and what problems he anticipated the two of them might have at some point in the future. He later became a psychiatrist, which, now that I think about it, might explain everything, but his "rational" way of choosing a lifetime partner drove me nuts.

"That's not really love," I told him. "You don't love someone because they meet the criteria on your scorecard; you love them because you can't help it."

In medicine, on the other hand, logical, rational thinking and use of statistics are rewarded. Medical schools teach that decisions should, whenever possible, be "evidence-based," and treatments are prescribed on the basis of controlled scientific studies that show those treatments to be safe and efficacious. In academia, any therapy that hasn't been proven in this way is scorned as "anecdotal," something to be avoided at all cost, and admitting that you are considering using an anecdotal treatment on your patient is on a par with confessing that you were abducted by Bigfoot while on a camping trip or that you secretly harbor a late-night bowling fetish.

This scientific approach to making decisions did not exactly come naturally to me. Growing up, I had always been more on the intuitive side, and highly sensitive – some would say overly sensitive – and slow to warm up to others. But if sensitivity makes relationships difficult, it also goes hand in hand with intuition and empathic understanding. I had learned early on in life that I could usually trust my gut feelings about a person or a situation, and that these feelings were rarely mistaken.

Then I went to high school and discovered that the people who were considered "highly intelligent" did not make decisions in an intuitive way; instead, they used reason and logic. This was an "aha" moment for me. I didn't want to be scorned as being "illogical" or "sentimental." I had always been a straight A student and I couldn't bear the thought of losing that identity. If intelligence was based on rational, Enlightenment-style thoughts and logical arguments, then I was determined to be the most rational person around.

Even though I had figured out how to get good grades, I still harbored the secret conviction that I wasn't really as smart as everyone else. I lived in fear of being unmasked as an imposter, like the villain in a Scooby Doo episode.

Medicine was not a field anyone in my family had previously entered. I had done surprisingly well on the Law School Admission Test and was strongly considering a career as an attorney – something I thought would be appropriate, given my lifelong love of writing and my propensity for mounting vigorous arguments in defense of my position on almost any issue. After impetuously signing up for a summer class on genetics, however, I decided that I wanted to apply to medical school.

When I left the liberal arts to study science, the rationalist philosophy that I had embraced in high school was strongly reinforced. Since I was taking all the prerequisites at once (human biology, organic chemistry, physics) I had no time to balance things out with a good Medieval Poetry class. Intuition was out; the scientific method was in. It was like discovering the keys to a secret clubhouse, where all the members were admired and praised just for being intelligent enough to find their way inside. I was converted.

Given this background and Cariana's diagnosis of Down syndrome, it was apparent to me that to cope with this problem, the thing I needed to do was to cobble together every minuscule scrap of information that was floating around out there and plan a rational response, based on the facts I had accumulated. I had lost control temporarily over the past few days, but researching options and analyzing data was something I knew exactly how to do.

I spent innumerable late nights at the computer, making lists and compiling massive amounts of information, all of which I painstakingly organized into a thick notebook with multicolored dividers, complete with subsections. This was in addition to ordering all the books ever written on raising a child with Down syndrome, every one of which I was determined to read before Cariana was six months old, just to be sure that I wouldn't miss out on anything I was supposed to be doing for her.

In medicine we have finally recognized that it is easier and cheaper to prevent illness rather than treat it. Patient education and disease prevention are now a large part of every primary care physician's practice, and preventive medicine has even become a specialty in its own right. This public health approach has worked, to some extent, for chronic diseases such as heart disease, asthma, and diabetes, considerably decreasing the morbidity and mortality associated with these diseases.

Child development is similar to medicine in that many problems can be prevented or ameliorated, especially if children receive support during the critical early period of development from birth to age three. In pediatrics, we spend the majority of our time doing "well child" visits, which many people think of as just being centered around immunizations but which, in reality, are important screening tools for evaluating each child's development. If we suspect any problems or delays, we refer that child for Early Intervention services.

Early Intervention therapists are the most loving and accepting people I have ever met. I imagine they are a lot like angels, except they wear pants instead of flowing white robes because they sit on the floor playing for most of the day. They somehow manage to see the amazing, unique potential in every baby, no matter how "disabled" that child may look to the rest of us. In the months Cariana had been receiving Early Intervention, I had learned much more from her therapists than she had.

Through our local Early Intervention agency Cariana received weekly visits from a developmental specialist, an occupational therapist, and a speech therapist. They interacted with her and, even more importantly, gave me tips on what I could do to help her during her "activities of daily living" – which, at the time the rash occurred, consisted mostly of looking at books, feeding herself, playing the piano, chatting on her toy telephone and scooting around the house. Everything the therapists did with her seemed like play, but it was all carefully designed to help Cariana reach her full potential.

Probably her favorite therapy was the horseback riding. When she was eighteen months old, she started weekly riding sessions with Challenge New Mexico. The horse's movements beneath her were supposed to teach her body how to balance and eventually walk; Cariana's favorite part, however, was being the object of so much affection from the people who rode with her and walked beside her. The workers and volunteers all seemed to look forward to seeing Cariana, and she returned the compliment, beaming at them and waving as we pulled up in our car. Friendship was not on the list of "benefits" to be gained from this particular therapy, but to Cariana, it outweighed all the rest.

The one thing all the therapists agreed on was that Cariana followed her own timetable, which basically meant that no matter how much we "worked" with her on something, she would wait until one day when she finally decided she felt ready and then show us that she could do it perfectly, as though she had secretly been practicing all along while the rest of us were sleeping.

Her developmental specialist once remarked that Cariana was constantly surprising her and the other therapists by mastering things they did not think she could do and refusing to do other things that they thought her body seemed ready for. Standing, for example, took her a lot longer than many other children, but she fed herself tidily with a spoon and fork by fifteen months of age, and she could point to twelve different body parts by name when she was only one and a half years old.

"Cariana took me to a deeper place," said her occupational therapist, "regarding what I thought I already deeply understood, summed up by the phrase, 'You can't push the river.'"

I couldn't wait for Cariana to start speaking, because I always had the feeling that she had a great deal of undisclosed wisdom that she was excited to share. Julie, Cariana's speech therapist, once sent me a beautiful letter about the lessons Cariana had taught her. She wrote, "Cariana did not speak any words for a while, but when she did, they were as clear as if she had been saying them for years. This," she added with considerable understatement, "does not fit the speech mold." I wasn't surprised, though; Cariana had never fit into any mold.

I discovered an entire world of therapies for Down syndrome. Besides the traditional physical, occupational and speech therapies, there was oral motor therapy, dolphin therapy, hippotherapy, patterning, cell therapy, and music therapy, not to mention a whole host of supplemental hormones and vitamins that were promoted as greatly reducing the genetic effects of Down syndrome. It was mind-boggling.

Like many other parents of children with Down syndrome, I threw myself into therapies with abandon. I was determined to make every minute count and make sure that no possible learning opportunities were wasted. Surely my daughter would be the exception to the rule, the "superstar" of the Down syndrome world who would meet all milestones early, defy all her therapists' expectations and leap tall buildings with a single bound. I was constantly talking to Cariana, naming everything in sight, teaching numbers and colors and shapes in the grocery store, singing the alphabet song to her in the car.

Cariana probably thought I was a bit crazy, but if she did, she never let on; she simply cocked her head and smiled at me indulgently with laughter dancing in her eyes. I suppose she somehow knew I needed more time to learn the lessons she seemed to have been born knowing. Lessons such as how to stop worrying so much about the future; how to feel my own worthiness, without having that feeling depend on my accomplishments or my productivity or whether or not I'm invited to join a certain book club; and how to slow down and truly enjoy each precious and unique moment.

It was so hard not to worry though. Worry is the heart and soul of parenting, even when your child hasn't been given a life-threatening diagnosis. When you are pregnant, you feel like everything you do could have far-reaching consequences for your child's future. The paranoia is fueled daily. You receive warnings everywhere you turn – from the nightly news, from the neighbor who stops you on the street, from magazine clippings your mother sends you in the mail: hair dye, cell phones, shellfish, acrylic nails, hot tubs…the list of possible teratogens seems endless.

When you finally have the baby, you stare at him in his crib, worried he will go to sleep and never wake up. You worry that he will never learn to walk, and then when he does, you worry he will trip and fall down the stairs and break his leg. You childproof the entire house but still worry he will somehow eat paste or pry the little plastic covers out of the electrical outlets.

When he goes to school you worry that his lack of armor makes him too vulnerable to be out of your sight. You worry that he won't have friends; and then when he does come home talking about the friends he made, you worry about what he will learn from them. Then your children become teenagers, and the worries seem almost endless: alcohol, drugs, eating disorders, smoking, driving, pregnancy, crushed dreams, broken hearts.

These were the kinds of concerns I had with my first two children, but when Cariana came along, I discovered a whole new set of things to worry about. When you are the parent of a disabled child, the worries are a hundredfold greater. Barbara Gill writes in *Changed by a Child* about something she calls the DIF equation:

> The normal tasks and frustrations of parenting are multiplied and amplified. Everything is at a higher volume,

> and there's more of it.... The actual incidents and events involved in raising a child with a disability are not, taken one by one, so different...from the incidents and events that are part of raising any child. The difference is in the Duration, Intensity, and Frequency of these events.... Other kids break an arm or have a serious illness; our daughter has had at least one surgery every year of her life.... Other first-graders have a teacher; ours has two teachers, a case manager, two paraprofessionals, a speech therapist, and an adaptive phys-ed teacher.

It's not that caring for a child who has a disability is always difficult – in fact, it's an amazing gift. But it does add an extra dimension to all the daily activities of life. It also changes you in ways that you could not predict or imagine. I feel a little sorry now for all the people who have never known this gift of raising a "special" child, a gift that forces you to slow down and ultimately makes you much more grateful. You don't put up with superficialities any longer. You appreciate everything because you know there is a razor's edge between joy and sorrow.

When they are newborns, some children with Down syndrome have such subtle features that the diagnosis isn't always obvious to strangers. As the children grow, however, there is always a point where it becomes more readily apparent. Cariana was born with very few of the usual stigmata—no crease across her palm, no heart disorder, no feeding difficulties – but I knew it was only a matter of time before she would have to go out into the world and face people who would judge her based on her facial features or her unclear speech or her unusual gait.

My biggest concern was whether people would see her Down

syndrome features and automatically assume she had whatever arbitrary limitations that person's life experiences had taught them to associate with that diagnosis. Initially I didn't really want to tell anyone she had Down syndrome. I was afraid she would suffer from what has been called "the soft bigotry of low expectations."

I wanted Cariana to have the same opportunities that other children had, without being judged prematurely. I knew that even if her abilities in certain areas were similar to those of other children her age, many people would not give her the benefit of the doubt or spend the time necessary to discover what she could really do.

While she was in the Early Intervention system, she would be encouraged and validated in everything she accomplished; but the public-school system is another entity altogether, and despite the advances in "inclusion" in recent years, all children still encounter the truth that a teacher's expectations lead to self-fulfilling prophecies. This has been borne out in many excellent studies: students do better when their teachers expect them to do better, regardless of their innate abilities.

Most parents end up worrying for nothing. Their children grow and thrive, and the things they fear never come to pass. But for me, the worries were no longer abstract; they were terrifyingly real. My child had been given one of those diagnoses that everyone fears, and with all my medical knowledge–after years of medical school, pediatric residency, and private practice – nothing I knew of could spare her from what was to come.

In an article by Dr. Brian Skotko, published in Pediatrics (Jan. 2005), almost 3000 parents of children with Down syndrome were asked how their physician had delivered the diagnosis and what their feelings had been when they were given the news that their child had Down syndrome. Although those parents almost universally saw their children as a blessing in their lives, the vast majority of the 1250 parents responding to the survey reported being told very little from their physicians about the positive aspects of Down syndrome.

There were stories of physicians blaming parents for refusing testing that might have allowed "early termination" as well as a report from one mother whose geneticist showed her "a really pitiful video…of people with Down syndrome who were very low tone and lethargic-looking, and then proceeded to tell us that our child would never be able to read, write, or count change."

This is one of the biggest problems with the medical model: it is deficit-based rather than strengths-based. It looks for what is broken and needs to be fixed, what is abnormal and needs to be cured. It sees every diagnosis as a problem to be solved instead of a unique attribute belonging to a person who is already perfect and worthy of being loved and included. It does not understand that every person has unique gifts and innate dignity, and each life adds something of value to the world.

Several prenatal screening tests for Down syndrome have been developed. The most significant part of all of these tests is that they are all promoted as providing answers sooner and faster. I know from discussions on Internet listservs that these types of news stories sadden many parents of children with Down syndrome. What does it say about our society that we have chosen to put the majority of our research money into tests that can detect Down syndrome and other genetic causes of mental retardation earlier and faster, rather than into research that would help people with those conditions to grow and learn and develop to their fullest potential?

I understand that parents want to know as much as possible about the health of their baby before that child is born. The part I'm afraid is at risk of being lost, in the rush to develop all this new technology, is that a test result is meaningless unless it is accompanied by honest, accurate information. True choice ought to mean an informed choice, and sometimes legitimate, factual information seems very hard to come by.

Most of the time in medicine, we hold to the fundamental principle that each human life is of equal value. When a patient is brought into the Emergency Room, the nurse doesn't hand them a multiple-choice questionnaire to evaluate their worthiness. The patients are triaged based on who is sickest; not who is the most likely to be able to sing the National Anthem in front of 30,000 baseball fans without utterly embarrassing themselves.

Outside the hospital, however, we do make these kinds of judgments. Instead of embracing the conviction that each of us deserves equal medical treatment, many Americans question whether they should be required to pay for the health care of the alcoholic whose liver is failing because he refuses to stop drinking, or the smoker who develops lung cancer, or the little girl whose parents willingly chose to bear a child with a disability, all of whom can be counted on to consume more than their "fair share" of the national budgetary pie. It is not particularly reassuring to remember that not so long ago, hospitals all over the United States routinely withheld medical and surgical treatment from babies with Down syndrome who were born with complicating conditions.

Life-saving treatment was withheld, at least initially, from Sandra Jensen, a thirty-five-year-old woman with Down syndrome and a congenital heart defect that eventually deteriorated to the point where, in 1995, she required a heart-lung transplant. Despite the fact that she had been living independently in an apartment in Sacramento for fourteen years, holding down a job and paying taxes, Stanford University Hospital and the University of California, San Diego both denied her the transplant, stating that people with Down syndrome are not "appropriate candidates" for the surgery. This conclusion was based on the assumption that a person with Down syndrome such as Ms. Jensen, who reportedly had an IQ of 70, would not be able to follow the complicated medical regimen required after the surgery in order to prevent rejection of the transplant.

Sandra Jensen's plight was taken up loudly by the media and subsequently, in 1996, Stanford agreed to perform the operation. She later died from lymphoma, which is one of the possible side effects of the immunosuppressant drugs taken after transplant to prevent organ rejection, and which was unrelated to her Down syndrome. In an interview before her death, she said of undergoing the transplant, "It's not for everybody…but I was asking them to look at me as an individual. And I think each person needs to be looked at as an individual."

If we deny life-saving medical treatment to certain individuals based on their disability, how do we avoid falling down the slippery slope to saying that they do not deserve to live at all? If we try to draw that line, we must realize as we do that the "disabled" are not some separate race living in a far-off country with impermeable borders. They are our parents, our children, ourselves. If a person's worth is conditional on appearance or ability, then everyone is at risk. Any one of us could become disabled tomorrow and suddenly be deemed worthless.

No test can tell us who our child will be or what gifts that child might bring into the world. Maybe we all could stand to be reminded that merely seeing an analysis of someone's chromosomes tells us next to nothing about the person herself, and that the effects of having three copies of the twenty-first chromosome are extremely variable and can in no way be predicted by a blood test.

Many people would have classified Cariana as "aberrant" and "imperfect". In our society, where it has become acceptable to judge another person's quality of life, many people – including some physicians – continue to question whether a person with Down syndrome can truly live a "quality life."

But Cariana, even as a two-year-old, had a higher quality of life than anyone else I've ever known. She sparkled with joy and sprinkled it like glitter onto everyone around her. She had a way of finding joy in the present moment, as if every minute of her life was a precious treasure. She enjoyed every day, she gave and received love every day, and she laughed every day – something most of us only aspire to but never achieve.

Cariana could stand by herself but wasn't yet walking, so to get anywhere she either scooted or, as happened most often, was carried. Unlike most children her age, she hadn't abandoned the affectionate baby stage and still loved to be held and hugged, which was perfect as far as I was concerned. Whether we were reading books, watching a video, or playing a game, she was almost always in my arms.

She never had a special object like a blanket or a bear that she was obsessed with. As Placi often said, "Cariana is only attached to you, Mommy." Her all-time favorite position of comfort was to be held against my chest, like a newborn, while she gently played with my hair. Whenever anything happened that upset her, I always knew I could calm her again just by picking her up and allowing her tiny hands to touch my hair; it never failed to soothe and console her. But what I had never fully realized before was that holding her also soothed and consoled me.

For years I had lived with the feeling that I never quite fit in anywhere. But Cariana and I fit perfectly together. Taking care of her was my ideal vocation; we each needed exactly what the other one had to offer. Cariana was kind enough to overlook my many failings and disabilities. She simply loved me, not for my grades, or for my appearance, or for what I could give her, but deeply and unconditionally – exactly the same way that I loved her – and we basked in each other's love like two cats stretching out in a warm patch of sunlight. And I slowly began to accept that if she was perfect just the way she was, maybe I was too.

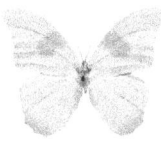

~Practicing Medicine~

Even after we knew Cariana's diagnosis, it didn't mean we had all the answers. In fact, we had more questions than ever. What would happen if Cariana didn't tolerate the drugs? How would we know if the treatment was working? What would the long-term cognitive or developmental effects be? None of those questions were answered to our satisfaction, either in the written protocol or by the oncologists. It seemed the more questions we asked, the more ambiguity we encountered.

Patients often think that having a diagnosis means their period of uncertainty is over. What they don't realize is that there is still so much that is unknown in medicine; even when we have a name for something there is no guarantee that we can predict the outcome or even come up with any adequate treatment. Physicians know this, but we also know that we have to make decisions somehow, with the knowledge and information we have, however imperfect.

We can gather the best information available and share it with our patients; we can give them excellent advice, based on our knowledge and experience. What we can't do, unfortunately, is give patients the absolute certainty they desire. This uncertainty – in making diagnoses, in choosing treatment options, in our ability to predict the outcome of those treatments – is the reason that medicine is still considered an art, even in this highly technological age.

On the other hand, sometimes when we have to deliver terrible news, we wish there was more uncertainty. My worst day as a pediatrician was the day I had to meet with the parents of a young boy in my office and tell them their son had a renal tumor. He received treatment and is doing very well now; but at that moment, I would have given anything to be able to tell them that I was really sorry, but I honestly didn't have the slightest idea what was causing his abdomen to protrude like that. I couldn't help empathizing with the parents and thinking about my own children.

We all look for compassion and empathy and understanding in our doctors. That's certainly what I wanted as a patient and the mother. But compassion, while necessary, is a double-edged sword. It can make us more effective as physicians, but it can also lead to depression and burnout. It takes an emotional toll when you constantly put yourself in another person's shoes, especially when that person is sick, or in pain, or dying.

It starts early in residency. There are so many patients, and so much work to be done, and we are taught early on not to get overly involved in our patients' lives. Connecting on a personal level with patients is usually seen as unprofessional - and even if it wasn't, there's no time to hold a patient's hand, no forum for expressing our sadness about the patients who are suffering and dying.

There is an element of pure self-preservation here that can't be avoided. If physicians truly put themselves in the place of every parent and every patient, they would all become overwhelmed within a few months and run away to some tropical island to make puka shell jewelry and rent out fishing boats. But cultivating too much detachment takes away from one of the true rewards of medicine: getting to know people intimately and learning the details of their lives.

I couldn't imagine how hard it must be for the oncologists to see so many children and families suffering, to give their hearts to sick children knowing that some of them would die. Most of them had children too; I could understand why they wouldn't want to get too close. But I still couldn't help wishing that they would come by our hospital room more often and talk with me longer.

Medical training is intense, high pressure, and intolerant of mistakes. In medical school I thought all the surgeons were arrogant, but later I discovered that wasn't true. It's just that surgeons have to be exceptionally confident; if they weren't, they would never be able to pick up a scalpel. They know as well as anyone that the science is inadequate and their skills, no matter how practiced, are still imperfect. But they have to be decisive even when they don't have all the answers.

It is often said that July 1st is the most nerve-wracking day to be a patient at a teaching hospital, because all over the country the interns – who were medical students just a week before – are starting their new jobs. As students, they had no real authority in the hospital. Days later, with M.D. after their names, they are able to write orders, prescribe medications, and admit patients to the ward.

Interns in July are learning their way around the hospital and are instantly recognizable by the "deer-in-the-headlights" expression on their faces and the bulging pockets of their immaculate long white coats. Back in the dark ages before smart phones, my coat had been heavily weighted down with books and notecards that I desperately hoped contained every bit of information I would need to care for the seemingly endless list of young patients that had been assigned to me.

One of my strongest memories is of my first time on call as an intern, after performing a particularly inept lumbar puncture procedure late at night. I had wanted nothing more than to crawl under the counter of the nurses' station to conceal my tears. I couldn't imagine how I was ever going to learn everything I needed to know. "Everyone is afraid of making mistakes," my senior resident told me. "You just have to hide it so you can function." I had been a doctor for two weeks; I felt utterly unprepared for the weight of the responsibility.

This inability to know enough or read enough isn't confined to medicine. It's everywhere we turn. I'm sure I am not alone in feeling completely overwhelmed by the sheer volume of information in the world today. It seems exponentially larger now than it did when I was reading my way through the Encyclopedia Britannica set in my living room as a child. My lists of "saved to read later" articles, movies and shows to watch, podcasts to listen to, books to read, and classes to take are impossibly long, and still I add to them every day.

When I entered medical school, I thought there was an enormous, but finite, body of knowledge that I needed to master. This was a fallacy. No matter how much you study, no matter how long you have been a doctor, there are always new medicines being invented, new procedures being developed, new research to be assimilated. There is always too much to learn and not enough time in a day to learn it all.

Dr. David Hilfiker writes in *Healing the Wounds*:

> I knew I was a 'good doctor.' Feedback from colleagues and patients was positive. But I recognized that in a wide variety of areas I was continually getting in over my head. My response to this situation was insecurity and self-doubt. I suspect other physicians may respond to similar

stresses by becoming excessively compulsive or overly authoritarian, but the situation itself cannot be avoided. As physicians, we are constantly confronting our own ignorance.

We don't talk about these fears openly enough. We talk about how "stressed" we are, as if the work itself was to blame. The dilemma is that nobody wants to think of their doctor as insecure, or in over her head. Atul Gawande points out in The New Yorker that "If the bell curve is a fact, then so is the reality that most doctors are going to be average." But as patients, we all want to feel that we are getting the best possible care, the best possible advice. We want to live in a Lake Wobegon world, where all the women area strong, all the men are good looking, and all the doctors are far above average.

This pressure to be perfect is the dirty little secret in medicine. Rarely, if ever, will anyone admit that they feel that pressure, let alone that they are affected by it, but we see the consequences of it everywhere we look. Burnout is rampant and increasing numbers of physicians are leaving medicine or retiring early. Doctors have the highest suicide rate of any profession, as well as some of the highest rates of divorce, depression and substance abuse.

Partly, this is because medicine attracts people who are perfectionists. It's what gets us through the long years of schooling and the sleepless nights of residency. It's also part of what makes an excellent physician. At some point, most of us come to the conclusion that the pursuit of perfection is a futile exercise. But coping with that knowledge is another thing all together, especially when you're trying to deal with the painful realization that your mistake might have seriously harmed a patient.

I don't know about you, but I make mistakes every day. I trip on things that aren't there; I over – or under-cook dinner; I wear mismatched socks. I've even been known to go into the grocery store and leave the car running with the keys in the ignition. Once I went a whole day with my shirt on inside out and backwards. These could be considered inconsequential gaffes, but medical errors are even more difficult to come to terms with. We have much more practice with defending our actions than we do with admitting our errors.

There are a lot of gaps in medical education. We are not taught how to accept our own fallibility, or how to deal with loss or death, or how to trust our patients. Patients want to be believed when they report something they feel is abnormal, and not have their opinions dismissed even when they may disagree with something that is common medical practice. And we often fail in that regard.

In *The Anatomy of Hope* Dr. Jerome Groopman relates the story of his colleague Dr. George Griffin, who was Chairman of the Department of Pathology at Harvard when he was diagnosed with stomach cancer. This type of cancer has an extremely poor prognosis. But even though all the other specialists caring for him thought the cancer was incurable, Dr. Griffin insisted on undergoing an extremely aggressive regimen of surgery, chemotherapy and radiation – which ultimately did cure him, though only after he endured excruciating side effects.

He knew the other Harvard physicians thought that he was either crazy or in tremendous denial. None of them believed that the surgery or other treatments would be worthwhile. As Dr. Groopman puts it, "I and the rest of the clinical staff had written George off. He would not be alive today if our recommendations had been heeded." As I read the book, curled up next to Cariana in the hospital, I was struck by Dr. Griffin's response:

> I knew all the arguments made in cases like mine. Treatment would cause unnecessary suffering – for me and for my family. Add in that it throws away society's money on a doomed person. I find these arguments patronizing…. Most patients don't really understand what's happening to them, how poor their prognosis is, because they're not clearly told the odds by their doctors…. I, of course, had a crystal-clear understanding of my chances. And it was my right to choose what I did…. I deeply wanted to live, so I had to fight.

Dr. Griffin's colleagues honored his requests for treatment despite their reservations, because of his status as a physician. But I couldn't help thinking that if another patient had asked for the same thing, they would have been denied the radical therapy, or at least strongly discouraged from pursuing it.

We don't always trust our patients to make decisions, to follow through on instructions, or to know what is best for them. Sometimes we are right, and they really don't take the medicine, or they really don't understand the situation. But we often forget that there are other ways of making decisions that have nothing to do with medical degrees or textbook knowledge.

When Cariana was in her sixth month of treatment, she was running high fevers, what is called "fever of unknown origin." Her doctors and nurses were all very surprised when the culture results came back: the bacterium that grew from her central line was a streptococcus species, the very thing we had been giving her daily penicillin to prevent. "Well, that just shows you that the prophylaxis [penicillin] doesn't always work," said Cathy, one of Cariana's favorite nurses.

This struck me as a good example of the way in which we, as doctors, make assumptions about our patients and their families. In this case, Cathy was taking for granted the fact that I had been giving Cariana the penicillin in the correct dosage every day. Because she trusted me to do what I was supposed to do, she concluded that the medicine had failed to work.

But I remembered many times during my residency when similar events had occurred with patients – when the medicines we prescribed either for prevention or for treatment of infections didn't seem to work – and the usual assumption of both the attending physicians and the residents was that the parents, who in that hospital were mostly of lower socioeconomic status, had obviously not been "compliant" – that they had skipped some doses, or had not gotten the prescription filled, or had misunderstood the directions, or in some other way had failed to follow our instructions.

I wanted to run back to Phoenix and track all those people down and apologize for not believing them. We had jumped to the conclusion that the parents had somehow failed, rather than accepting the possibility that the drug had failed to do what it was supposed to do. We had trusted the medicine more than we trusted the people.

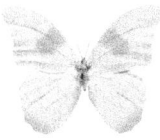

~To Hope or Not to Hope~

All three of our kids loved dancing to music, but they each had a different favorite song. Placi liked to sing – or rather shout – all the songs he learned on the playground, including "He's a jerk, he's a bore, no more purple dinosaur," and the current favorite going around the school, "Jingle bells, Batman smells, Robin laid an egg." Liesl's favorites, on the other hand, consisted of the classic "Blah Blah Black Sheep" and Paul McCartney's famous hit, "Band on the Sun."

No matter how many times I tried to tell her the correct lyrics she refused to believe me, which I suppose is not really so surprising when you consider that denial was becoming a way of life at our house. You had to keep on believing what you believed, because admitting things could be otherwise was unimaginable.

When caring for patients with life-threatening illnesses, the hardest part of a doctor's job is deciding when to continue to offer hope and when to suggest that further treatment is not in the patient's best interest. The best doctors, the most adept, are able to combine both options, somehow suggesting that the patient or family may want to consider stopping treatment while still holding out some semblance of hope. I've heard rumors that doctors like this exist, the way the Loch Ness Monster has occasionally been sighted, but no one has ever been able to provide any proof more substantial than a blurry photograph.

We struggle to accept that we cannot save a patient, especially when the patients are children. In a survey of 122 emergency physicians cited in the 2002 Institute of Medicine report on pediatric end-of-life care, more than two-thirds admitted to prolonging resuscitation efforts in order to delay telling parents their child had died.

Communication is always fraught with possible errors. We think we have explained the risks of treatment, or the chances of survival, but the patient or family may have an entirely different interpretation of the conversation. In a Yale University study, 69 percent of the terminally ill patients who were questioned said their doctors did not discuss their prognosis with them, although the doctors reported they had done so. I can tell you from experience that half of what was said to me in those critical conversations went right out of my head seconds later.

I kept asking Cariana's doctors for explanations, but I think deep down what I really wanted to ask them for was hope. Some days, when the blood counts went up, they seemed to give it; other days, not so much. She would improve temporarily, then slide backwards. One day she would eat well, the next she would barely drink. She lost weight. She looked tiny and fragile. Though I refused to feel hopeless, I did frequently feel helpless. There was so little I could do.

What I could do, and did, often, was pray. And so did everyone else. We were a non-denominational cause: Catholic family members prayed for us; Jewish friends prayed for us; Presbyterians, Lutherans, and Methodists prayed for us; even a Muslim family, who were friends of friends, prayed for us. The thought of all those prayers offered me some hope, and I clung to it the way Liesl clung to her Teddy Bear, desperate to believe that it was real.

A recent poll reported that almost half of all Americans said that they pray or meditate every day. But even though I prayed myself, I couldn't keep the question from forming in the back of my mind: were all those prayers actually doing anything?

In my copious free time, when I wasn't occupied with more important things such as napping, I looked for an answer to this question and found that there was a whole body of research on prayer that I had never heard of before.

Several studies on the power of prayer published in the Archives of Internal Medicine, the Journal of Reproductive Medicine, and the American Heart Journal all seemed to show that praying for someone at a distance did have a beneficial effect, even if you didn't know the person, even if they didn't know they were being prayed for. The Heart Journal study, for example, involved 150 patients who were scheduled for angioplasty with stent placement. They were randomly assigned to one of five groups: guided imagery, stress relaxation, healing touch, off-site prayer, or no complementary therapy. None of the patients, family members, or staff knew who was being prayed for, yet the "prayed-for" group had fewer complications than any of the other groups.

Now I could think of a lot of potential problems with this kind of research, not the least of which is this basic question: How could the researchers ensure that the people in the "control group" were not, in actuality, being prayed for by other people uninvolved in the study – say, for instance, their mothers?

The most interesting thing about all this research was that the prayers that seemed to be the most effective weren't prayers asking for a specific outcome like praying for a tumor to disappear. The most effective prayers seemed to be the ones that were non-directive, when the person praying simply asked that whatever happened would be "for the best." But I struggled to apply these studies to my own situation. I knew exactly what I wanted to pray for. I honestly felt that I knew what the best outcome would be in this situation, and I wasn't about to stop hoping that we would get it.

Sometimes people ask me why I go to church. In the course of the conversation, it usually turns out that these people used to go to church, but left years ago for one of two reasons. Either they decided they could not tolerate what they saw as hypocrisy, or they were angry with God over some painful event in their past when their prayers seemingly went unanswered.

I understand this feeling, but I still pray most days. Even though I almost never get a direct answer, somehow praying helps anyway -- maybe because the act of praying reminds us that we are part of something greater. Praying in a church, or any group setting, is powerful because it makes us feel connected to something larger than ourselves.

We obviously don't need to go to church to find God. God is just as present in the grocery store or a forest as in a cathedral. We go to church not only to find God but also to find ourselves there – the self that is able to pray, to connect, to listen. And to find others from whom we can gain encouragement and comfort.

One of the reasons I love my church is that there is room in it for people like me – people with questions, people who don't fit in. We have members who are committed to the faith even though they are not theologically literate, and we have members who are extremely theologically literate and still admit to suffering crises of faith. The people in my church don't fear the questions. They understand that faith is not a coat we put on but a series of stages through which we struggle.

I have been friends with four wonderful Presbyterian ministers in my life – Robert Rounce, Sheila Gustafson, Matthew Davis and Harry Eberts – and I have asked them all, at various times, the same question: "Why should we continue to pray, to hope that we will be heard, when so many times our prayers seem to go unanswered?" And they all gave me basically the same response, that essential tenet of Christianity that says we really do receive an answer to our prayers, it's just that it isn't necessarily the answer we were praying for. We pray for one kind of healing and we receive another. We pray to change the world (or a test result) and instead we find that we ourselves are changed.

But the one thing no one has ever been able to explain to my satisfaction is the verse in the Bible where Jesus says, "The Father will give you whatever you ask of Him in My name." As I said, I don't claim to be a religious authority, but I just don't see the wiggle room there. It doesn't say if you ask for one thing you will be given another thing that's better for you, like a child who goes Trick-or-Treating for candy and is given some toothpaste or maybe a carrot. It says whatever you ask for will be given.

I tried believing that whatever happened would be for the best, but that Panglossian philosophy simply didn't ring true; there was only one outcome that would be "best" as far as I was concerned. I just couldn't bring myself to believe those people who kept telling me "Things may seem bad now, but they will make sense later on," or the always popular "Everything happens for a reason." Cariana's illness didn't make sense, and there was no good reason for it.

It's not that I don't believe in God. I have felt the warmth of an overpowering love. I have no doubt there is a force in this universe that is much greater than my mind can comprehend, and I have certainly seen many instances of alchemy in my life, where something beneficial and even beautiful somehow flowered out of the rocky soil of pain and despair.

But that only proves that good can come from bad. It doesn't necessarily follow that the bad thing occurred purposefully so that the good thing would result. I couldn't believe everything happens for a reason because to me, there was no "reason" that would be good enough to justify what was happening to Cariana. Whatever good might come of it, to me it would never be worth the price.

Miracles have been documented often enough that I really do believe they occur. A malignant tumor mysteriously vanishes, a woman survives a fall off a cliff, a blind man wakes up able to see. St. Peregrine, in the fourteenth century, prayed the night before he was scheduled to have his cancerous leg amputated. He dreamed that Jesus came down from the cross and healed his leg, and when he woke the next day the cancer was gone and never returned.

If I had no faith at all I could scoff at these stories and call them coincidence. My problem is that I do believe God can work miracles. What do you do, then, with a God who can perform miracles and simply chooses not to? Thomas Merton wrote "Suddenly there is a point where religion becomes laughable. Then you decide that you are nevertheless religious." Maybe the biggest miracle is the fact that we continue to hope at all.

In the 1840s (and even today, in some circles), many people believed in faith healing. If a person was healed, it was felt to be because of the healer's powers combined with the strength of the sick person's faith in God. If a person wasn't healed, it was because they had insufficient faith. This was the perfect setup for the faith healers. They couldn't fail, because failure was always the sick person's fault.

But what if no one is at fault? Is the randomness of fate really so intolerable that we have to see causality everywhere?

At our local Catholic high school, they pray before every

sporting event, and plenty of people would be quick to tell you that the reason they won the basketball game by one point in the last three seconds of overtime is that God was on their side. But do we really believe that a God who would help a basketball player sink a free throw would refuse to intervene to save a child's life?

I wanted to shrug off despair like a sweater. I wanted to be blasé and insouciant about the whole thing, to move confidently onward, smiling serenely, like my childhood hero Nancy Drew would surely have done. But it was simply impossible. The knowledge that the chemo had failed to work gnawed away at the edges of my hope, leaving it as bedraggled as Placi's fraying blankie.

Amid the constant din of what I thought was a successful life – studying, working, achieving, parenting – it had been impossible to really hear myself. When I was forced to be quiet and still, holding what was most precious to me in my arms and knowing at the same time I might lose her – only then could I start to listen to the voice that had been trying to speak to me all along. At this point, though, what I heard from the inner voice was mostly fear. I was terrified of running out of options.

Self-help books often talk about "letting go" as if it is always a good thing. But that's an oversimplification, because letting go isn't always the answer, and it definitely isn't always appropriate. The truth is, there are some things we aren't supposed to let go of. Things like hope, and love, and memories.

I refused to give up hope, but it seemed to be slipping away anyway, fading gradually like a Polaroid picture. I was basically living in a hospital; they should have been able to help with this dilemma. If I was losing blood, I could get a transfusion of someone else's blood to replace the blood I lost. But what can they do when you lose hope? Do they have other people's hope stored in jars somewhere so they can replace mine?

My usual response to impending doom had always been to imagine the worst-case scenario and preemptively prepare my defense against it – but that strategy failed completely as I faced the possibility of a life without Cariana. There was no way I could prepare for that.

Part Two

Today my world is ended
My heart no longer sings
I fold my pride about me
As angels fold their wings

-Pearl S. Buck

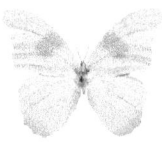

~A Grief Observed~

April 2004:

Life, it turns out, is a lot like a funeral. There is deep sadness, and loss, and pain; but there is also love, and gratitude, and laughter, and food. Specifically, casseroles.

Several nurses and doctors attended Cariana's memorial service, including Becca, one of Cariana's favorite nurses. Afterwards, she took off her own silver bracelet and gave it to me. It said, "And Lo, I am With You Always." I wear this bracelet every day now, as it seems to me a message not just from Becca, but from Cariana as well. The woman I see in the mirror each day looks stiff and pale and painted slightly, like the people in old photographs. I've become extremely susceptible to waxing poetically on depressing subjects. Also to a variety of airborne viruses. According to family lore, my great-aunt Minnie wore black for seven years after her son drowned in the early 1900s. Aunt Minnie, if you're listening, I completely understand.

I can scarcely bear to leave the house because everywhere I go, I keep seeing eerie doppelgangers, as if there is a convention in town of little two-year-old blonde girls with pigtails. But I can't stand being home either. Even with her bedroom door closed, everything reminds me of Cariana: the stool she used to perch on, the high chair where she would sit and laugh at me while I cooked; the kitchen still stocked with her favorite foods (macaroni and cheese, spaghetti, sorbet).

It stuns me to see life going on around me, people shopping for clothes, riding their bikes, going out for dinner, buying stamps. My daughter is dead! The world should have come to an end; the earth should have stopped rotating on its axis.

It's nice to think that everyone in a family will pull together in their time of need, but what happens more often is that each family member is floating on his or her own raft, too far apart to even reach the others. We don't want to add to each other's suffering, and we are each so consumed with our own pain that it's almost impossible to help anyone else. All I really want to do is crawl into a cave and hibernate, like a bear; but unfortunately, even though I can hardly help myself, other people are depending on me to help them.

My pain seems to seep up continuously from some bottomless well, relentless and unstoppable. I have no idea what to do with it. I expected the emotional numbness, but what I didn't expect was how exhausting grieving is. Every day I try to run, but my legs feel as if they've been filled with lead. I feel wrung out, used up, spent. All I have inside are leftover emotions, like the broken, sad detritus of a summer yard sale.

Last week, in the early, pre-dawn hours of the morning when I was half awake, I suddenly realized I was holding something warm and heavy and very familiar in my arms. My happiness was indescribable. Every day I had prayed, over and over, "Please, just let me hold her one more time." And now my prayer had been answered. I refused to open my eyes, afraid the sensation would disappear. I just lay there for what seemed like hours, savoring every precious second, until at some point the weight lifted gently and was gone. Everyone tries to console me by telling me that I took such good care of Cariana, but I know the truth: she was the one taking care of me all along, and now she was doing it again, reaching out with love to comfort me and soften my pain.

The other day I took Placi and Liesl to the car wash where we are frequent customers. The girl behind the counter asked innocently, "Where is your little girl?"

"She died two weeks ago," I told her softly.

But that doesn't really answer the question, does it?

I refuse to say I lost my daughter. I didn't lose her; she was taken from me. The question of who took her haunts me.

Did God take Cariana away from us? Did He cause her illness? I have never believed that God is the cause of all the pain and suffering in the world, and I don't want to start now. I don't blame God because I can't bring myself to believe God caused – or chose - Cariana's death. I can believe that God created a world in which human beings, microbes, and cancer cells exist, but I can't believe in a God who chooses specific individuals to suffer from one disease or another.

God doesn't spend the day helping our team win the World Series or finding us parking spaces. Bad things happen even to people who have strong faith. "Trust in God, but lock your car," as the bumper sticker says. I don't believe God wanted Cariana to get leukemia or wanted the 9/11 passengers to board those planes. I do believe God uses whatever there is – including crises and suffering and the brokenness of the world – to open our minds and hearts. I don't believe God caused Cariana's suffering, but I do believe God suffers along with us.

Some Christians I know like to say that God never gives us more than we can bear. But if you look around any city or read any newspaper, you find multitudes of people who were given more than they could bear. Depression, alcoholism, substance misuse, addiction, toxic stress, suicide: all are evidence of people who were crushed by the weight of having to bear the unbearable.

May 2004:

It's late May, but all the calendars in the house are still displaying April. I start flipping through the pages of the calendar, whiting out doctor's appointments and coffee stains with fervor. If only they made whiteout for life, so we could erase the parts we didn't want or need anymore. I wake up most mornings to a split second of normality, the sun on my face; but it's always followed by a sickeningly fast roller coaster descent as the cold, hard truth slaps me in the fact again: Cariana is gone.

Placi and I checked out a library book written by Jane Goodall two weeks ago and we're finally getting around to reading it. As we huddle under the covers, I read aloud Jane's description of the way in which chimps grieve for each other. One chimp, an eight-year-old named Flint, was with his mother, Flo, when she died; afterwards, he seemed lost, not wanting to eat or interact with the other chimps, as though he simply couldn't cope with life without his beloved mother. He died six weeks later.

"I think he died of grief," Jane wrote.

Placi looks at me with worry welling up from deep in his brown eyes. "Will we die of grief too, Mommy?" he asks.

"No Buddy," I tell him as I hug him tightly. "It only feels that way."

Liesl, only four, looks at things differently. She has her own way of hurting, but she has no developmental framework with which to understand the permanence of death. She often asks me how long Cariana will be gone, or when we will see her again, as if she is impatient for her to return from an overextended vacation. She doesn't want to sleep alone, however, and every night gives her a new chance to create ingenious excuses for why she can't possibly stay in bed.

One thing she doesn't have trouble with is talking about Cariana; in fact, Liesl seems to be the only family member who regularly brings up Cariana's name in conversation. When the pest control service man came to our house, Liesl followed the poor guy around, distressing him by relaying unwanted news such as "This was my sister's bedroom. She was two and she died," or "This chair is where Cariana used to eat – before she died," or even "This is where our cat is buried; her name was Penny and she died right after Cariana."

Liesl needs someone to lie down with her, something that has become routine. She crawls into bed beside me, her face still painted from her visit to the Children's Museum earlier today.

"Can I tell you something Mommy?" she whispers.

"Of course, sweetheart."

"I hope this doesn't hurt your feelings," she says, touching my wet cheek. "I want to cry about Cariana, but I just can't. I'm sorry."

"It's ok, honey," I tell her. "You'll cry when you're ready. And if you don't, it's ok too." Then I add, "I'm sorry Mommy keeps crying. It's just because I wish Cariana was still here."

"Oh Mommy." She looks up proudly, her eyes shining. "Cariana isn't gone; she's just gone into my heart!"

June 2004:

My friends have no idea what to say, because, of course, there isn't anything to say. Nothing that will really help. Nothing that will bring real comfort or consolation.

"She knows you loved her."

Yes, she does, but she didn't have to die for that. She knew I loved her when she was in my arms too.

"She is at peace now."

Yes, I believe that, but she could have been cured and still continued to live in peace.

"She had a wonderful life."

Yes, she did, but she deserved a much longer one.

"She loved you so much."

Yes, but that knowledge is so intangible. So much of love is related to touch. It's the way we connect with each other, the way we give reassurance and affection. Abstract love, the memory of love, is vaporous and ephemeral compared to the feeling of my child snuggling in my arms.

July 2004:

I had one job – to protect my child and keep her safe - and I failed completely. It's easy for me to believe that the doctors and nurses did their best, but much harder for me to accept that there wasn't something I missed, something I could have done. I have many flaws – impatience, shyness, a well-deserved reputation for choosing bad movies – but I've always been a big believer in second chances and pretty quick to forgive others. The only person I have trouble forgiving is myself.

I'm bombarded almost daily by subtle suggestions that perhaps I could use a teensy dose of medication. It's amazing to discover how many people in our society see medicine as the answer to every ailment – as if any medicine exists to treat this kind of pain. We live in a "fix it" world: cut it out, take a pill, fix whatever is wrong and move on. If we can't cure it, we quickly become uncomfortable with it.

Luckily, I have two wonderful therapists who know the difference between depression and grief. I'd like to try to explain it to the Prozac-pushers, but I hold my tongue because I understand their motivation. They want to see me happy again so they can feel better. My sadness is a constant reminder to them that the things they fear the most are the very things they can least control. They don't want to face the fact that anyone might die tomorrow, even people we love fiercely and passionately, even people for whom we would give our own lives.

August 2004:

If April was the cruelest month, August is the saddest. Today, August 6th, is the one-year anniversary of Cariana's diagnosis, and the memories of that terrible time have flooded back clearly and painfully. It will also be her third birthday at the end of the month. And it's the month Placi and Liesl will return to school, reinforcing the fact that my status as full-time-mother-with-little-children-at-home-who-need-me is officially over.

On August 29, Cariana's birthday, we bring flowers and balloons to the cemetery, where the highly decorated "children's row" can be seen from the road as we drive by. Each gravesite holds colorful flowers, pinwheels, and toys left by those who came to mourn the small child who brightened their lives so briefly. I stop here twice each week, once to pick up everything before the mowers come through, and again the next morning to replace it all. Occasionally I run into another mother doing the same thing farther down the row. I wonder if we should form a club, like people do for books or wine.

I go home and sit in Cariana's room, looking at the crib where she used to peek at me through the wooden bars. I stare at her yellow fleece blanket printed with pictures of smiling children and her favorite toy, a musical phonics radio. I hug her pink and purple flannel pants, folded neatly on the closet shelf, and hold her little white shoes up to my face. I cry until my eyes burn and my chest aches.

Grief, I have learned, does not really lessen with time. It becomes papered over by daily life but it's always there, just waiting for some trigger that tears off the paper and exposes it again: the sight of a little blonde girl in pigtails; an article about a child with Down syndrome; an anniversary; a glimpse of a photograph.

In the office where I write, I sit and stare and the three beautiful faces in frames on my desk. Two of the faces in those frames will continue to change, adding new pictures on top of old, year after year. And one will not. One face will be forever two years old, with sparkling eyes and pigtails and two missing teeth.

September 2004:

It's the third anniversary of the September 11th tragedy, and the papers are full of articles on grief. Interviews with widows and children, analyses of the psychological effects of grief, expert opinions on the nation's ability to rise above our collective fear and become stronger through our mourning.

Lying awake again in the middle of the night, I congratulate myself on how far I've come. I sleep in a bed most nights now, instead of fully clothed on the couch, so that's something. Also, I no longer stand in the kitchen eating chocolate frosting out of the can; now I've graduated to Ghirardelli squares in colorful foil wrappers. This last accomplishment seems to me a huge step, like being promoted from Bear Cub to Webelo Scout. I should invite some friends over to celebrate; the only problem is that I can't think of anyone who would be happy to be called at two in the morning. I need to find a new group of friends – all night taxi drivers, possibly, or the waiters and waitresses at Denny's.

The bandages, syringes and oxygen tubing still tower in the corner of the living room, taunting me, along with a pair of tiny flowered hospital-issue pajamas. If I give the hospital back their pajamas, will they return my daughter to me?

October 2004:

Placi and Liesl are both on soccer teams, an activity that takes up four afternoons per week. And then there is the therapy – individual therapy, group therapy, couples' therapy. You name it, we're doing it. In addition to seeing the school counselor every week, Placi and Liesl have their own child psychologist to talk to, and they are both attending after-school groups at Gerard's House, a center for grieving children.

Strictly speaking, this may be more therapy than is absolutely necessary. Then again, I suppose some people would look at me and argue that it's clearly not enough. One bright side is that the hectic family calendar is probably saving me from attempting to drown my sorrows. If I started drinking, I would undoubtedly overdo it and be encouraged to attend Twelve Step meetings, something I definitely don't have room for in my schedule.

While the children meet at Gerard's House, the parents and caregivers meet too, in their own space, and a bond of understanding quickly forms. The support group is comforting in a fraternity sort of way: we share a secret, and we all live in the space between anniversaries, and for many of us, this group is the only place we really feel free to open up.

Each meeting seems to develop a theme of its own as the discussion goes on, and this week several people report a similar phenomenon – looking everywhere for their loved ones. A young woman in mismatched clothes says she always looks around the mall for her father. A graying father with sad eyes looks in crowds for his daughter's red hair. A fortyish, dark-haired Hispanic woman describes calling her mother on the phone to borrow a jar of spaghetti sauce. Only after the phone rang several times did she realize there was no one there to answer it.

The first annual Grief Index, compiled in 2002 and reported in the *Wall Street Journal*, suggests that grief in the workplace carries a hidden cost of over $75 billion. I think the grief literature – in which I've become an unwilling expert – has a lot to teach us about life in general. People grieve differently, they say; there is no one right way to grieve, no set amount of mourning time that is right for everyone. In our "regular" lives we give lip service to the idea that everyone is unique, but how would the world be different if we truly adopted that idea and accepted it completely, the way grief specialists do?

Acceptance and validation are difficult for people who have never experienced this kind of grief. Not even the people closest to me can feel what I'm feeling or truly understand the depth of my pain. Even in a family, even in a marriage, every person has to bear their own, specific grief. No one else can inhabit this world with me.

Part Three

Verily you are suspended like scales
between your sorrow and your joy

-Kahlil Gibran

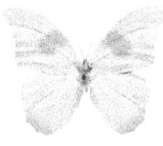

~Growing Pains~

Grief is a journey, and the biggest gift anyone can give to friends who are grieving is to let them choose their own path and then simply travel with them along the way. My path was introspection through reading and writing. In my grief, I turned to my old childhood friends, books, and they didn't let me down.

Nature abhors a vacuum, so the space the lost one leaves behind has to be filled with something. Some people fill the space with work or sports or other activities, scheduling time for everything except the grief itself. Sex after a funeral is a commonly used trope in literature, a way for the grieving to reaffirm that they are still alive, a way to feel something again besides just emptiness and pain. It all works for a while, but in the end, the grief is still there, lying in wait underneath the rug, until eventually it trips us up when we least expect it.

Reading and writing filled the space for me. It is what I do, what I have always done, and it comes as naturally as breathing. Reading is inhaling, taking in stories and metaphors and meaning; and writing is exhaling, pouring out the emotions that need release. It is also helpful that reading and writing are both solitary activities. I didn't want to hide from my grief. I wanted to immerse myself in it, to experience it to the fullest and be transformed by it, and somehow, I sensed that transformation would require stillness and solitude.

We sometimes fool ourselves into thinking that all of life can be sorted out and categorized neatly into boxes: physical, emotional, spiritual. What no one tells you is that sadness – pure, deep, untouchable sadness – is not just an emotion; it's an actual, physical pain. Mothers who have lost a baby frequently report that their arms continue to ache for the child they cannot hold. My whole body ached to be with Cariana, aghast at what had been ripped away.

I've been told that to say, "I miss you" in French the expression is "tu me manques" which literally translates as "you are missing from me." I can't think of a more perfect way to express the sense of loss. It's not just that I miss her voice, or the touch of her hand on my hair; it's that a part of my own body is gone. There is a hole in my heart, a Cariana-shaped piece that is missing.

In *Hallucinations*, Oliver Sacks wrote about the experience of having a "phantom limb". He described people who continued to feel the sensation of a physical arm or leg even after it had been amputated. Sacks quoted a French surgeon, Ambroise Pere, who noted, "Long after the amputation is made, patients say they still feel pain in the amputated part…which seems almost incredible to people who have not experienced this." The idea did not seem incredible at all to me. Because Cariana had never learned to walk, I had carried her everywhere. My arms could still feel the weight of her physical presence, cuddled next to my chest, and being without her did feel like an amputation.

I have always felt as if I don't quite belong in the world, as if I was accidentally dropped off here by mistake. As a child this fact made me feel isolated and alone. Spending time alone, however, isn't always a bad thing. It's especially useful for me as a coping mechanism given the fact that I find large groups of people very stressful.

In recent years it's become more commonly known that introverts need time alone to recharge their batteries, but when

I was growing up, I never heard of that concept. All I knew was that the continual interaction demanded by school, friendships and family relationships was a constant source of discomfort and struggle.

When Cariana died and my world fell apart around me, I needed solitude more than ever. The stress of daily living was so great that I didn't have any energy left to give emotional support to anyone other than my children. My tendency to retreat into my shell when I feel overwhelmed has contributed to the failure of at least two serious relationships in my life. Retreats are nice, if you use them as a restorative to prepare to come back into the relationship. But if you stay there too long you might find you have no one to come back to.

By mid-life, most people have had at least a passing encounter with sorrow, but I had suffered more losses than most, including my father, my mother, my baby daughter, all four of my grandparents, and eight aunts and uncles. Not to mention all the very real and significant losses that come with divorce: loss of identity, companionship, status, family and friends.

People sometimes tell me they find me surprisingly optimistic (usually followed by the unspoken "considering your child died" facial expression, accompanied by a sympathetic head nod.) But as a child I didn't feel very optimistic, probably because I was easily overwhelmed whenever I encountered pain or sadness. I can't watch the news, because when I hear a report of a teenager committing suicide, I feel a stabbing pain of despair and hopelessness. I can't watch *Game of Thrones*, because seeing the trauma the characters go through traumatizes me. I can't go to an animal shelter to play with the dogs, because I don't just see the sadness and longing in their eyes, I actually feel it.

Those of us who grew up being ridiculed for being "too sensitive" know that our culture does not do well with people who feel deeply. In my high school yearbook, a friend wrote, "You need to make your sensitivity a strength instead of a weakness." Sadly, many people don't see sensitivity as a strength. They want the sensitive folks to medicate those messy feelings away and "put on a happy face." But it seems to me if your heart isn't broken at least once a week by what you see in the world, you simply aren't paying close enough attention.

Being alone was my one safe haven - especially being alone in my own home, which I had deliberately crafted over the years to provide that comforting feeling of safety and peace. I love how Cheryl Strayed describes it: "Alone had always felt like an actual place to me, as if it weren't a state of being but rather a room where I could retreat to be who I really was." I had no idea how to put my life back together, how to find meaning and purpose and a new way of living. I was just trying to keep from breaking down in sobs while passing the baby food aisle in Albertsons. In my heart I knew I had to go to that "Alone" room. I had to sit in stillness in order to figure out who I was in light of this loss, and who I wanted to become.

Sitting quietly and just waiting had never come naturally to me, but having a sick child had been a crash course in learning to wait. Waiting for test results; waiting for appointments; waiting for the doctors to make their rounds or for the medicine to start working. I didn't know it at the time, but I suppose, in a way, all that waiting was preparing me for all the waiting that was to come: waiting for guidance, waiting for transformation, waiting for a new life.

Surprisingly, I found that when I was sitting in the waiting room at the pediatric oncology clinic, the waiting area itself felt to me like a sacred space. The waiting room felt as holy as a chapel in some ways, a place of intimacy and raw emotion, where honesty was everywhere because everyone in the room understood there was no time for anything less.

We are a culture in love with busyness and productivity. We fill all our blocks of time with meetings and sports and social commitments. We feel like we always have to be "doing something". We now have an epidemic of people sitting in their cars at stoplights while texting or looking at memes or sending photos to friends on Snapchat, because we can't stand to just be still, even for thirty seconds.

Lately, it seems that whenever I ask someone "How are you?" the most common response by far is "I'm so busy". We almost seem to take pride in being able to say we don't have any openings in our schedule. We think if we are not busy, we are doing "nothing." But sitting in stillness is not the same as doing nothing. It's how we learn to listen.

The problem with keeping our calendars so full is that there is no white space, and the white space is what we need in order to process our pain, transform and grow. Over-scheduling keeps us too busy to think, too busy to feel, and gives us plenty of distractions from the things we prefer not to deal with, like that bothersome grief. The true self is heard only in silence and the din of modern life easily drowns it out. But even in the midst of non-stop media chatter, it's still there somewhere inside, nagging at us, lying in wait for a quiet moment. In silence, we learn to trust the voice inside that tells us the truth when we are still enough to listen.

The busyness numbs the pain the same way people use food, or drugs or sex. And it works, right up until the moment when we are unexpectedly still for a few minutes – on the subway, perhaps, or in church on Sunday morning, when the pain unexpectedly seeps out of the corners of our eyes during the Pastor's sermon. This happened to me not infrequently at First Presbyterian Church of Santa Fe, as my body took advantage of the one quiet moment in the week when I was forced to sit still and be present-- the one quiet moment when the cries of my heart could be heard.

I have always been ambivalent about going to church. This is perhaps reflected in the fact that I am never on time for any church function. Somehow, though, I felt as if church had something I needed, so I kept attending in spite of the tears it frequently triggered. Out-of-town visitors often looked at me strangely, while the regulars exchanged knowing glances as if to say "There she goes again." I took to hiding pocket-sized tissue packets in the back of the pews so I could surreptitiously wipe my eyes while pretending I was searching for the One Great Hour of Sharing envelope.

It's awkward to have your emotions broadcast to the world like that, which is why we usually hide them. We stuff our feelings down with ice cream and potato chips; we numb our brains with vodka martinis; we work late into the night and take online classes and schedule meetings on weekends just to ensure we don't have time to sit and think. We do all these things because they make the pain tolerable and they make us more comfortable. Which is why the distractions don't get us anywhere. Because real progress, real transformation, is by its very nature uncomfortable.

Life gives us that lesson over and over. There is no birth without pain. There is no rebirth without death. There is no transformation without some sort of loss. Over and over, life teaches us that we have to risk losing something in order to become something more.

I'm not saying I like this. I would much prefer to have the growth and transformation without the pain and loss. In fact, it's one of the things I really want to ask God about, if I get the chance, right after "Why did Cariana have to die?" and "Really? 108 years? Think of all the Cubs fans who died waiting!" But, in my more rational moments, I have to admit I do see some possible value in setting up the system this way.

My friend Harry, who is also the Pastor at First Presbyterian Church in Santa Fe, pointed out one Sunday morning that God always chooses the people who don't seem up to the job. God didn't choose the smartest, or the most spiritual, or the most popular people to carry His message. He chose the outcasts, the sinners, the flawed human beings like Jacob and Saul and David, because those were the people who were most in need of transformation.

We can grow without experiencing a painful loss, of course, but it certainly makes change easier when you have that kind of catalyst. When we're knocked down flat on the ground, unable to move, we're finally still enough to hear our own true voice. Transformation doesn't always mean a huge, outwardly visible change, like giving up a job, or a relationship, or making a cross-country move. But it always means losing one thing to gain another. And often, what we need to lose isn't a job or a place or a person, but an attitude or belief that is keeping us stuck.

It's painful to shine a light on these attitudes and really look at ourselves. Many people go their whole lives without attempting it. (As Tom Hanks said in "A League of Their Own", "If it wasn't hard, everyone would do it.") Transformation isn't necessary to live, of course, or even to be happy. A caterpillar could be perfectly happy living its whole life as a caterpillar, never knowing it was meant to be a butterfly. But transformation is definitely necessary if you want to grow and blossom and become the full person you were meant to be.

Transformation is part of the classic hero's journey, a common theme in stories through the ages, from the ancient Greek myths to *Star Wars*. According to Joseph Campbell, this is why myths are so enduring and so powerful: they're really about the spiritual quest to find the authentic "you". In the end, he says, we find and meet our destiny not through technology or even through reason, but by getting in touch with our own inner being and discovering the resources of our own character.

It is possible to fake transformation of course. If we choose the right words, post the right pseudo-spiritual quotes, and present our story in a carefully curated, Facebook-friendly way, we can seem openhearted and enlightened without going through the gritty work of actually transforming. Real growth takes time, not the six months most people are willing to give us. You have to feel your way back. You can't research it, reason it, or logic your way through it.

The seed that is planted by the gardener must feel as if it is dying when it is being buried in the earth. But that "death" is necessary for the plant to bloom in the spring. We hold on through our pain, through what often feels like a painful death, because we know in our hearts we are more than the body we inhabit; we are a soul trying to bloom. And experience tells us that even though some winters last longer than others, the spring always comes. We build fires, and we knit blankets, and we light candles, and we make cocoa. And we wait for the sun.

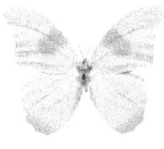

~Signs of Life~

I have very few memories of my childhood and high school years, possibly because I spent so much time just trying to navigate through the world that I wasn't paying much attention to anything else. It always makes me laugh when people talk about how they find it difficult to stretch beyond their comfort zone, because practically everything I do in my daily existence is outside of my comfort zone. There are so many people, so much information, and so little space and time to make sense of it all.

Organizing and scheduling and making lists all help to contain the chaos. But I still come home drained at the end of almost every day. It takes constant focus to be present and listen to others, which I find exhausting.

I once read a book whose author described two types of people: those who fill your bucket and those who drain it. I've definitely known people who made me feel drained if I spent any significant amount of time with them. Time with my children, on the other hand, always fills my bucket. My favorite thing to do is laugh and joke with them. When they were small and always with me, I was perfectly happy having them as my closest friends. Okay, maybe they were my only friends.

Other than my children, it's rare for me to find someone I truly feel comfortable getting close to--which probably explains why I have so much trouble letting go of those rare, special people when I do find them. Unfortunately, we can't surround ourselves only with people who energize and restore us. Most of us have to come in contact with a wide range of people every day, many of whom are only too happy to tell us who they think we should be and what we should be doing with our lives. Society at large, from TV ads to social media, constantly tries to tell us who we are.

But the answer to that question ("Who am I?") can never come from anyone else; it has to come from our own inner voice, which is often the hardest to hear. So much of our daily stress comes because we are living everyone else's plans for our lives and not our own. When we're feeling confused, it's been my experience that it usually means we feel torn between what our true self is whispering and what the outside world is telling us we should do.

When we find the right people, or the right path, the ones that resonate and support us in being our true best selves, we usually recognize those things, because the joy is unmistakable. When we don't recognize those things that are meant for us, the lack of recognition, I believe, is usually due to fear.

Fear blocks the signals, like aluminum foil blocking radio waves. If we are afraid of starting a relationship, or taking a new job, or of making any kind of commitment, then our fear will blind us to the signs pointing us to those things, even if those signs are right in front of us. If you're not even asking the questions, it's unlikely you will understand or even notice the answers.

And the answers often don't come as clearly or as quickly as we would like. Sometimes we have to just sit with the questions, and that is something that's difficult for many of us. We are addicted to the quick fix, the easy solution. Instead of waiting to go to the doctor, we Google our symptoms and get answers in 1.3 seconds. It doesn't seem to matter whether the answers are true, or scientifically verifiable, just as long as they are available quickly. Want spiritual growth? Better intuition? Serenity? Inner peace? Just download the right App and it can all be yours, without any struggle or waiting.

But guidance and knowledge and deep understanding don't work that way. They don't come quickly, and they don't always come in the form we expect. Frankly, I'm just as suspicious of those who find a quick and easy path to enlightenment as I am of someone who claims they have never driven over the speed limit.

I wanted guidance on what I should do with my life, because the possible consequences of making the wrong choice seemed intolerable to me. In the movie *Sliding Doors*, the main character, played by Gwyneth Paltrow, is shown in two different scenarios. We see her life play out completely differently based solely on whether or not she makes it onto a certain train. If the doors close before she can get on, her life travels on one path; if she gets through the doors and onto the train, her life path is switched to another track altogether.

This is paralyzing if you really think about it.

The saddest and truest statement I know is that everything does not happen for the best. It can't, really, because we aren't puppets, or computers running pre-programmed algorithms; we are human beings who have freedom of choice. And because we are human, those choices are not always for the best. We can and do make bad choices, and so can other people. And other people's choices affect us too, in ways we may not even be aware of. We could miss out on what might have been our greatest happiness due to a choice someone else makes, and we would never know.

I do think there are things that are "meant to be" in the sense that those things would be for our highest good. Those are the things that would put us on our best path, and that is the way we will be led if we ask for guidance. I believe there is a plan, but we are allowed to embrace or reject the plan, even to our detriment. That belief is why platitudes such as "everything always happens the way it's supposed to" have never resonated with me. It's also what keeps me up at night. Because if we are free to reject – or simply not recognize - our destiny, how do we move forward?

I always believed that God had a plan for me. But I was afraid I wouldn't hear the guidance, or I wouldn't recognize the plan, or I would mess up and use my free will to reject a gift that was right in front of me, and I would miss out on something great. Maybe there was something special I was supposed to do with my life, and I would mistakenly pass right by it. I was afraid of choosing the wrong fork in the road, or the wrong road altogether.

I knew I had to find a way to create some sort of new life, because the old life, the one that was focused around Cariana, was over. It just wasn't clear what that new life should be. Should I go back to work, sit in an ashram in India, sign up for tango lessons? I prayed for clarity, but it seemed elusive. Maybe, I decided, it was too hard to do this alone. I would look for someone or something that could help me discern the messages.

Discernment is about knowing when to act and when to wait. As in whitewater rafting, the time to act is when you are in the midst of the rapids. You don't have to paddle on the slow, drifting part, the guide tells you, but when things get rough, you'd better jump into action if you don't want to capsize. This is the exact opposite of what we want to do. When things slow down, and quietness envelops us, we get anxious. We want to get busy paddling. And when it gets rough, sometimes we are paralyzed with indecision and refuse to act at all.

In my quest for guidance I sought out anything and everything that promised to help me. Since I live in Santa Fe, there was a seemingly endless array of choices. A quick hour or two of research led to the discovery of numerous spiritual practices, all prominently promoted in books hastily borrowed from my church's library or listed on the back page of the Santa Fe Reporter, and all of which claimed they would assist me in listening to God, or my "inner voice", or my "Guides."

"Who knows what might help?" I shrugged. "Why not try them all?"

I visited a psychic medium, a Shamanic healer who was married to a Reiki specialist, two Spiritual Directors, and an Angel Whisperer. I practiced Centering Prayer on a church retreat, walked a labyrinth during a full moon, tried Vipassana meditation at a Buddhist Temple and attended a Christian Yoga class taught by a young Jewish woman who was annoyingly peppy. Whether the guidance came from God, angels, intuition or "the Universe" didn't really matter to me at that point. I was feeling completely lost, and I was looking for any signs I could find that would point me in the right direction.

I did see many things that I interpreted as signs from Cariana, things that warmed my heart. These are the sorts of events Jung referred to as synchronicity: meaningful interactions and coincidences that seem to defy linear causality and point us towards the spiritual plane of existence. Sitting at Placi's soccer game, a small boy with Down syndrome (whose family I had never met) crawled right into my lap and made himself at home there. Making home visits to hospice patients, my then-husband heard a dying woman describe being visited by a "little blonde girl with pigtails" who "sits on the floor because she can't walk", something that mystified the woman's family since they had no idea who the little girl could be. These types of signs were wonderful and comforting, but did nothing to direct me on what I was supposed to do with my life.

Honestly, I don't think I was asking for much – only a few brightly lit, gigantic neon billboards with unmistakable flashing green arrows. I find it extremely disappointing that God doesn't seem to visit people in burning bushes anymore. Spirit generally speaks in gentle whispers, like my grandmother used to do while she rolled peppernut dough in her arthritic hands and laid the little round cookies out on an aluminum cookie sheet in perfectly symmetrical lines. It was hard to hear her then, even when we were in the same room; it's almost impossible to hear the small voice whispering from the depths of one's own heart. That's why it only happens if we seek out the quiet spaces.

Over the centuries, seekers of spiritual transformation have always sought out those quiet havens. The ancient Celts talked about "thin places" where the veil between heaven and earth is lifted and God is closest to man, the places where the Spirit is near enough for the whispered message to get through. Harry described in a sermon a magical trip he and his wife Jenny took to Iona, Scotland, which historically has been regarded as one of those thin places and has been called the Birthplace of Celtic Spirituality. From their pictures, it's stunningly beautiful; however, we don't have to travel 4,539 miles to find locations that bring us closer to heaven. We have our own places of pilgrimage right here in New Mexico.

The Benedictine monastery in Abiquiu, Christ in the Desert, lies tucked away in the New Mexico landscape about an hour away from my house. It's completely invisible from the highway, and can be reached only by traversing thirteen miles on a rough, hilly dirt road. Despite this, the monks see a stream of visitors weekly, all searching for space and silence in which to seek and (hopefully) find God, and themselves. These visitors understand that when you quiet your mind and pay attention, you discover what brings peace to your soul, and what you can and cannot live with (or without).

When I first visited the monastery, it surprised me that so many people were interested in going on a retreat. I was a person who had always assumed more effort was the answer to any problem, so sitting quietly in silence did not seem to me like an effective way to search for answers. In the Midwest, where I grew up, there is a widespread belief that hard work is not only required, it's what makes the end result worthwhile. And this is true, to some extent. In general, I do think we value things more when we have worked hard for them. But there is also a time and place for giving up all our effort and just allowing ourselves to be open to what comes.

The silence provided by the monastery grounds us and serves as a rare respite from the cacophony of our culture. It strikes me every time I visit there, the immediate sense of wonder and stillness blending with the quiet of the monks' daily activities. This quiet is what draws people in. When the noise of the world is stilled, we can finally hear our own voice and see ourselves clearly. This is both exhilarating and terrifying, since most of us aren't sure what we will hear when we listen to our hearts. What I heard in the stillness was my desire to life a life that was meaningful, peaceful and connected to something bigger than myself.

We live in a world that prioritizes the rational over the spiritual. Intellect and reason and logic - these are great things. But reason and logic by themselves can't tell us the direction we need to go in order to find joy, or hope, or meaning. In quiet we can hear our inner voice, be guided by our intuition, and, if we're lucky, even receive some guidance from a higher power.

At least four times in my life, I have been blessed with that gift of guidance. The first time it happened I was given direction about where to go, quite literally. Driving alone from Denver to Santa Fe to start a medical school rotation, I got caught in a blinding snowstorm on a lonely and dangerous stretch of highway crossing the Raton Pass. If I had known anything about the Pass (or driving in general, really) I would never have attempted it. But neither of those things was true, so I drove on in a whiteout, oblivious to the danger.

I was running low on gas and couldn't see the lines of the road, let alone any signs of civilization. At some point I started to get a tiny bit worried and began to pray. Just then, a truck's taillights appeared out of nowhere right in front of me. Those taillights lit the road and guided me all the way into town, where the storm softened into gentle flakes as I gratefully filled my gas tank. Years later I drove it in daylight and was shocked to discover how steeply the cliff dropped off on the side of the road, which must have been only feet from my vehicle.

The next two gifts of guidance were job-related. In 2008, while in the process of finalizing my divorce and still grieving the loss of my marriage, I felt led to call an acquaintance, someone who had worked for the New Mexico Department of Health but whom I hadn't spoken to in several years. That call ultimately led to my job as Medical Director for Children's Medical Services, a program that serves children with chronic medical conditions and special needs. In that role I found dedicated colleagues who became dear friends and work that brought meaning and a sense of purpose back into my life.

The third message came a few years later when I got a clear feeling that I should apply for a promotion to run the Family

Health Bureau, a job that had just been vacated. The Public Health Division had never had a physician as the Bureau Chief before, and it required combining two positions, but doors opened and the needed support for the change materialized. Through that job I met some wonderful mentors and discovered amazing new challenges and opportunities for growth, and I think the Bureau has benefitted as well.

The fourth and most recent guidance I received was when I met someone who felt like home. I'm not talking about lust, or falling in love (although of course I did fall in love with him later.) "Home" is just the best way I know to describe the sense of total belonging I felt whenever I was with him. It astounded me, not only because the feeling was so strong, but also because it's so unusual for me to feel at home with anyone.

I was just recently out of an engagement and not at all interested in dating, having decided that I should probably start looking into solo travel, or perhaps adopting some nice shelter cats. But being with him felt like coming home after a long vacation: safe and comfortable and simply right in every way. Spending time with him gave me the same warm feeling of relief and gratitude I had felt that snowy night many years ago: the realization that this path, which had suddenly become visible right in front of me, was the one that would get me where I needed to go.

There were other signs as well - things I won't go into, mostly having to do with how we met - but suffice it to say that to me, the message that this person should be an integral part of my life was as clear and bright as a huge neon billboard. One of the fundamental features of billboards, however, is that they have two sides. And those sides often present two completely different and unrelated messages, depending on your vantage point.

Anyone who has taken a road trip knows that signs are easy to miss if you aren't paying attention. One person may notice a certain billboard, and another may drive right by without seeing it at all. If anyone had bothered to ask me, I would have suggested a much better system, where messages would come as a firm slap on the back of the head and the timing would always be miraculously right for both parties. This is the downside of "messages" and "intuition" – we have to be prepared in order to hear them. Like Brigadoon, they're only visible when the timing is exactly right.

I knew I needed to get to know this person as well as I possibly could, and to do it in an open and authentic way because that was the only kind of connection that felt right to me anymore. One of the gifts Cariana gave me was that she taught me how to love deeply and unconditionally. She modeled this kind of love – it radiated from her eyes and was felt by everyone who knew her. Compared to her I'm still a beginner at it, and I still mess up quite a bit, but at least I know what my goal is, and I feel as if I'm getting closer to living that kind of love with each passing year.

Grief also teaches that lesson about loving openly. When we deeply understand that any of the people we love could be gone at any moment, we don't want to be defensive or hold back anymore. In the beginning loss is isolating, but ultimately, we feel even more connected to others. There is a liberating fearlessness that comes from this hard-won knowledge of the fragility of life. When we truly grasp that this present moment is all we have, there is nothing left to do but give everything we've got, expecting nothing in return. We know our hearts will probably be broken, and we choose to love anyway.

Ironically, to the other person, a desire for deep connection can easily be misinterpreted as pressure. Which is why we have to meet people where they are. Connection can't be forced, any more than a bulb in the ground can be forced to bloom before its time. Living in an open, authentic way takes courage, because even when we take the risk and speak our truth, we may find that the person we want to connect with isn't ready or willing to open up to us. I felt sure we were meant to be together, not only because of the signs and the feeling of belonging, but also because of the way we brought out the best in each other. But he didn't see it. What seemed clear and obvious to me was foggy and unrecognizable to him.

There is no earth-shattering culmination to all this. I can't say I found an Oracle that gave me all the answers about what I should do to rebuild my life. But in a way, that's a good thing. Ultimately, I realized that looking everywhere for signs (and refusing to act or make a decision without receiving some sort of spiritual guidance) can become just another way of trying to convince ourselves that we are in control, when what is really required of us is to give up the insistence on control and accept that much of life is not within our control at all.

Searching for signs can also become a way of justifying inaction – a way to stall, or buy time, or an attempt to cover up our fear of making a mistake. And I should know; I'm the poster child for that strategy. I spent three years in Spiritual Direction, ostensibly seeking guidance but also, I think, seeking a reason to postpone making a necessary decision.

In the Christian tradition Spiritual Direction is an ancient ministry of the church in which a trained Spiritual Director assists an individual or small group of people in becoming more attentive to God's presence in their lives. It is designed to help us discern and become open to the will of God.

Our little Spiritual Direction group met weekly on Thursday nights, and we became very close over the years. I spent most of those weekly meetings with my minister and my fellow group members asking for guidance about a relationship I was in, but that guidance never came, at least as far as I could tell. I finally made the decision myself and ended the relationship, but it probably would have been better for everyone involved if I had done it much earlier.

I do think signs occur - to comfort us or reassure us or to help us know we are on the right path - and I still feel blessed when I receive those gifts of signs or a little help with discernment. I keep an eye out for heart-shaped rocks, and clouds shaped like angels, and the little yellow butterflies that will always be, to me, a sign of Cariana's presence. But I also know seeking absolute certainty is a fool's errand. Just ask the people who have thrown away thousands of dollars looking for guidance from inauthentic fortunetellers and fake psychics.

Luckily, even when we don't get the flashing neon sign we asked for, we still have our past experience to guide us. And experience teaches us that while loss is painful, it's also freeing. When we've gone through something wrenching and transformative it's almost impossible not to reprioritize our lives and how we spend our time. What used to seem so important now seems insignificant with the new perspective that loss brings. It's like stripping belongings from our backpacks on a long hike to lighten the load. We have to get rid of what's weighing us down, because it's the only way to move forward.

The truth is that when guidance does come it usually occurs in a completely unexpected and surprising way. This is amazing and wonderful, but it can't be counted on to occur when we need it or when we ask for it. We can spend our whole lives waiting for a "sign" that this is the perfect job or the perfect person. We can waste years waiting for the "perfect" time to act. Or, we can choose to take that step, make that decision, write that book, commit to that person in spite of our uncertainty.

Life will always be uncertain, uncontrollable, and unpredictable. We pray for guidance, and sometimes we do receive it. But we need to be careful not to use the search for guidance as a crutch to avoid taking action. Sometimes, all we can do is take a leap of faith, jump into the unknown, and hope for a soft landing.

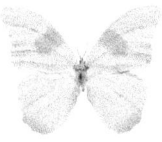

~Unexpected Gifts~

It would be great if living an open and authentic life meant everything else would miraculously fall into place. In an ideal world, people would think my authenticity was charming. They would offer me a prestigious award, or at least a nice fruit basket. They would feel safe with me, and they would share their story – their whole story, not just the whitewashed, socially acceptable parts. It's not impossible, and sometimes in the right circumstances this sharing can happen rather quickly. But more often it takes time, and patience, because sharing makes us vulnerable, and vulnerability isn't easy for most of us.

A friend and mentor once told me that friendship flows from vulnerability, because we connect more with people's vulnerabilities than with their strengths. If you want to make someone your colleague, he said, talk about your work and your ideas. But if you want to make someone your friend, talk about your most embarrassing moment, your biggest regrets, or your deepest heartache. There is a lot of truth in this, but it requires the right setting, and people have to be ready to hear those stories.

At Gerard's House, the people in my support group did feel free to be vulnerable. The best description of a grief support group I ever heard was that it is like a river that is always flowing. The people on the banks look at the people in the river and can't understand how they got there or how it feels to be in the water, being pushed along by the current. But three months from now, someone new will join the group (and be pushed into the river) even though right now they are completely unaware of what is coming. The river is always there, always running, buoying up those who find themselves there, helping to move us along so we don't stay stuck.

Pretending, like spandex, helps you look good on the outside, but it's always a relief when you finally take it off. I had specialized in defensiveness and self-justification in my past relationships, a reflection I think of the fact that it is so easy to feel criticized and so difficult to feel loved. But after knowing Cariana, I no longer felt the need to defend myself. I fully recognized that not everyone I met would like me, but that knowledge no longer upset me because living in an honest, openhearted way was more important to me than gaining people's approval.

I have a bit more courage now, especially when it comes to knowing myself deeply and being willing to share that self with others in an authentic way. Somehow being so completely loved by Cariana freed me from the need to be loved by others. I've been through the worst thing imaginable, so being rejected for a job or a book club doesn't seem like such a big deal anymore. Seeking approval always fails in the end anyway, because the finish line is always moving. Even if we manage to win someone's approval temporarily, it could be withdrawn tomorrow. One wrong word, one difference of opinion, and it can all disappear, like pulling one thread on a sweater and watching the whole thing slowly unravel.

Some people in my support group pointed out that losing their loved one had made them fearless, as if they had nothing left to lose. Of course, the truth is that as long as there is one person left in the world that we love, we still have something more to lose. But I think the point is that the future isn't quite as menacing after you have become deeply acquainted with grief. Things that used to seem terrifying, such as getting fired from a job, or speaking in public, or telling someone you love them, are nothing compared with what you have already faced.

One reason for this, I think, is that you have discovered your inner strength. I don't think we become stronger from suffering, because the strength was there inside all along; it's just that we were never sure whether if it would really be there when we needed it. If you have always lived a charmed life, you don't know what you are truly capable of surviving.

Another gift Cariana gave me was a feeling of connection with others. Sensitive people are often among the most compassionate, because they empathize readily, putting themselves in the other's place. But sensitivity does not necessarily lead to compassion or compel a person to help others. It can actually serve as a deterrent. Empathizing with everyone you meet is a difficult way to move through the world. Those of us who feel things more strongly have to work even harder at staying open and not shutting down to avoid feeling overwhelmed. I am easily hurt to the point of tears by what I witness in the world.

More than twenty years ago, neuroscientists studying monkeys in Parma, Italy noticed a strange phenomenon. They found that the monkey's brain contained a special type of cells called mirror neurons that fired in the same way whether the animal was performing an action or merely observing another doing the action. We now know that the human brain has many of these mirror neurons. When we see someone undergo something painful, our own pain areas of the brain are activated. We are, quite literally, hard-wired for empathy.

I think it's very possible that the more sensitive souls among us have more mirror neurons. For most of my life, my sensitivity made me want to withdraw rather than reach out, because I was continually being hurt by being rejected or excluded from one group or another. But sitting in the hospital room watching CNN for hours on end, I began to feel deeply connected to everyone else in the world that was suffering – many of whom, I freely admit, were in much worse circumstances than my own. The global pain that I had previously viewed from a distance suddenly seemed real and intensely personal.

Nature teaches the same lessons of the importance of connection and the importance of supporting each other. I love to hike on the weekends, and being out on the mountain restores my soul. I am reminded of these lessons every time I see the way the Aspen leaves shimmer in the breeze or the way the wildflowers grow with abandon on the hillside or the way the icy creek rushes in waterfalls down from the snowy peaks.

The mountains of Santa Fe glow with golden Aspens every October, a breathtaking sight against our bright blue skies, drawing visitors by the hundreds. Aspens are unique in that they grow in large colonies that can be derived from a single seedling, with new trees springing up from the spreading root system. The trees in the colony are all connected at the roots, sharing water and resources across miles of forest, and the roots can live on far after the individual trees have fallen. Like the Aspens, we are all connected to each other, all part of something much greater than ourselves, something that preceded us and will outlast our individual lives.

Water in New Mexico is a scarce and precious resource, and it must be shared. The water underground is tapped into by multiple individual wells, but they are all connecting to the same, shared source. The Rio Grande is tapped by farmers all along its route, from Colorado through New Mexico to Texas and into the Gulf of Mexico, connecting everyone who touches it along the way.

At the pool our family joined several years ago, the lost and found table always struck me as a perfect example of sharing within a community. The table is much more than just a repository of missing items; it is a resource, freely available to everyone. The people at the pool take what they need, use it for the day, and return it to the table. Towels, goggles, sunscreen, toys – whatever it is you forgot that day, you can probably find it on that table, waiting to be shared.

Ironically, meditating and praying – even alone and in silence – actually helps us feel connected with the world because it forces us to slow down and opens our hearts to greater awareness. But this awareness certainly doesn't have to happen in church. It can come from hiking in the mountains, or meditating, or watching the ocean rise and fall, or volunteering in a school or at a homeless shelter. Finding some way to feel connected to others is crucial, not only for our own sanity but to give meaning to our days and to our lives.

Eventually, like so many who suffer pain or loss, I turned to helping others. If I couldn't help Cariana any more, I could still help other children like her. Children with disabilities, children with cancer and other chronic medical conditions, children who were labeled or dismissed or not given an equal chance, children who were excluded on the basis of their chromosomes or their behaviors or their immigration status. That was the only thing that made sense to me and brought me some sense of peace.

I can only do very small things, but every day I am grateful for my job and the fact that it allows me to play this role. And every time I can do something for one of those children, I feel like I'm doing my own tiny part in helping to repair the world – "tikkun olam" as my Jewish friends would say.

It may seem contradictory to say that I have accepted that much of what happens in life is out of my control, while at the same time saying I am finding meaning in working to help others and repair the world. But I think those beliefs actually complement each other. Religions throughout the world have always recognized this. Pope Francis famously said, "You pray for the hungry. Then you feed them. That's how prayer works." Our hands are the hands of God. We are the way God works in the world.

We are meant to be here for each other, to share our lives, to support each other. Yet we are so busy we don't always make time to spend with the people we care about the most. My favorite thing in the world to do is just to sit and listen to the people I love tell me about their day. But I also know that for years, I was so overwhelmed with work and chores and "life" that I let some of those moments slip by. And when I am really honest with myself, I know that my greatest suffering has come from those times I felt disconnected – from the people I loved, from God, or from myself.

At a Down syndrome conference we attended in Denver when Cariana was nine months old, a speech therapist remarked in a lecture that in order to learn to communicate, what a child with Down syndrome needs most is a "focused and interested listener." When I heard that I thought, "Isn't that really just what everyone needs?"

I accept that suffering is an inevitable part of life, but I also think we should try to reduce that suffering. Feeling our own sorrow allows us to feel the sorrow of the world, and gives us the desire and the courage to work to alleviate that sorrow. Reducing suffering is a kindness that we should extend to others and ourselves whenever possible, because helping others is what we're here for. It is the outward expression of our deepest values, the ones that cross religious and ethnic boundaries.

We can't help everyone, but we can help the ones who cross our path, the ones who bump up against us, the ones who touch our hearts and whose pain keeps us up at night. And because we are all connected, any help we can give to any individual in our lives contributes to healing the world at large.

Part of that healing, in my mind, is working to make the world fairer. Of course life isn't fair; even children discover that very early in life. But we can make it more fair. We can work towards equity, and try to alleviate disparities. We can make it clear that when Black babies are dying at twice the rate of White babies, that is not something that is acceptable in our country.

We need to do our best to make the world fairer, not because life is fair but precisely because it isn't. Because unjustness in the world, I believe, is painful for God, and painful for all of us.

Things happen all the time for reasons that have nothing to do with what is "best"; in fact, a lot of things occur that are distinctly not for the best at all. Cariana developed leukemia because sometimes the cells in our bodies malfunction. Hurricanes and earthquakes strike because of weather and the shifting of tectonic plates. Relationships begin or end because of decisions made by others and events that are largely out of our control. Doors open or close for us because someone somewhere made a choice, and their choice affected someone else's choice, which affected my choice, and so on and so on. The ripple effects are endless.

It's easy to see how the "everything is for the best" theory got started. Psychologists tell us that humans have cognitive biases and seek psychological consonance: once we choose something, we have a strong incentive to believe that the outcome we chose is the best of all possible choices. Simply put, it feels good to think you have made the best possible decision, so we convince ourselves that our choice was for the best.

God's purpose for us is ultimately goodness. Perhaps what we end up with is not what was originally intended for us, but that doesn't mean it is second best either. I believe there is a plan for each us, but that plan is constantly evolving. If someone or something thwarts the plan, then God comes up with a detour.

Someone else may have locked the door we feel guided to walk through. So, we try again. We find another door, and another and another. And when one of us feels like giving up, others step in and help with the search. Which is why I am still optimistic about the human race. We regroup. We find new doors. We circle the wagons. We light fires and we build shelters and we keep each other warm.

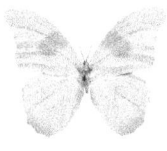

~Alchemy~

In 2015 I read a book called *The Life-Changing Magic of Tidying Up*. The author, Marie Kondo, helps her clients declutter their homes (and lives) with what has come to be known as the Konmari method. Basically, it upends the usual way I would "declutter" which would be by looking through my closets and pulling out things I thought I could give away. With the Konmari method, it's not so much about deciding what to give away as it is deciding what to keep. You pick up each item and then make a deliberate decision to keep only the items you truly love, the ones that "spark joy."

The method did help me simplify my home, but I think the more important lesson is the way it can be applied to life. Ms. Kondo herself points out that when her clients declutter their houses, they often find they can't help but declutter their lives as well. Perhaps this is because the process is tied closely to one's emotions. You know what to keep because when you hold it, you feel joy. It's really very similar to using your intuition to know whom you belong with, or what job you should take. What's right for you will feel right and bring you peace.

A postcard I had taped to my computer monitor at work for years reminded me daily to "Find the Joy." Partly, finding joy comes from taking time to develop self-knowledge and self-awareness, because these qualities actually help plant the seeds for a more joyful life. Joy comes when we share our true selves and our gifts with the world, and you can only do that when you know who you really are.

People sometimes ask me how I learned to laugh again. They want to know the solution to the sticky problem of grief. They want a back-up plan, a list they can keep in their pockets in case they experience grief at some point in the future, like the way my son's friend Damian keeps a "bug-out bag" in his truck packed and ready to go, filled with freeze-dried rations and lots of small ammunition.

Ten years ago, I would have had that list ready for prospective grievers. In fact, I did start a list back then, in 2006. It was called "How to be Happy," and it included the following: 1) write down your story; 2) remember what you still have to be grateful for; 3) focus on helping others; 4) find small moments of joy; and 5) when all else fails try a margarita. With the possible exception of the alcohol, all of these things have been scientifically proven to boost happiness.

I eventually came up with a more detailed list of "100 Things that Bring Me Joy" which I kept in my phone and referenced frequently. The list reminded me that no matter how hard a day (or a year) might seem, there are still many things in the world that do make me feel joyful, and the vast majority of them are small, seemingly insignificant things. Things like watching a beautiful sunset, listening to ocean waves, the feel of soft kitten paws or rabbit fur, a cozy room lit by candles, putting on pajamas warm from the dryer, or cooking with my mother's 50-year-old pans.

At the risk of sounding like a cliché, I also started keeping a gratitude jar. When something funny or surprising or amazing happened – or merely something that brought a smile to my face – I would write it on a scrap of paper and drop it in the jar. Pulling those papers out later and reliving those occasions magnified the gratitude even more.

These things served me well at times when the sadness seemed overwhelming, reminding me that there were still many ways to find some happiness, or just moments of peace, even on the worst of days. But the real answer of how to survive loss and grief can't be boiled down to a checklist or a pithy quote. It's about opening your broken heart and letting in light and air to heal the broken pieces. And opening a broken heart is both the simplest and the most difficult thing we do.

Mindfulness, like gratitude, is an over-used word nowadays, but it really does help us to open our hearts. Mindfulness is not the same as meditating, something I have attempted on multiple occasions but still struggle to do for more than thirty seconds. It's simply about cultivating the ability to notice the small moments of beauty and to fully embrace those moments by paying attention.

In this age of multi-tasking it seems almost sacrilegious to talk about focusing on only one thing at a time. We shower while listening to the news, we make dinner while watching Netflix, we make phone calls while driving in the car, and I am as guilty of all this as the next person. But I also know when I do those things that I am not giving any one of those items the attention it deserves. As the Vietnamese Buddhist monk Thich Nhat Hanh puts it, "While washing the dishes one should only be washing the dishes, which means…one should be completely aware of the fact that one is washing the dishes."

I still tend to multitask most of the time, but I've found that fostering this kind of single-minded focus when possible really does help keep me from rushing around mindlessly, missing the joyful moments altogether. Most importantly, I intentionally apply this lesson when I am spending time with a person I really care about, giving them my full attention and focus, and this one action has done more to improve my relationships that anything else.

The oncologists had a saying about living after a child dies: "You either get bitter, or you get better." Loss will change you; there's no way around that. But how it changes you is up to you.

It is only with time that we eventually learn that grief cannot be controlled any more than illness could, or death. Our attempts at controlling grief do nothing more than bury the pain so we can pretend that we have "moved on." At this point we have two choices: we can keep the grief buried and move on with our well-planned lives and our to-do lists; or we can let the grief surface, let it flow over us and wear us down, like water wearing away a rock and polishing it all at the same time. This is the lesson of acceptance. When we finally and completely accept that we are not in control, when we give up that illusion and the false self that goes along with it, then we are able to truly become someone new – our real Self. It brings us to a more honest place, where everything is stripped away except for love.

There is devastation in our world today, but there is also goodness and resiliency and generosity and beauty. We hear stories of people who have lost everything, who have endured floods and earthquakes, wildfires and hurricanes, and who, in spite of their own suffering, step up again and again to assist others. There is still much to have faith in, even when our prayers aren't answered.

Maybe that is the real purpose of grief, to break us down and make room for those other things we need in our lives. By having a capacity for so much grief, somehow it enlarges your capacity for joy at the same time, so that eventually they can exist side by side. The grief never leaves, but somehow it also makes room for the joy.

I see both the beautiful side and the dark side of life, and how they coexist, the same way laughter and sadness coexist in me. It's what the Franciscan Priest Richard Rohr calls "bright sadness," what the Japanese refer to a "mono no aware," which means something like "a sensitivity to the pathos of things" or "beauty touched with sadness." Perhaps this has been the most profound lesson of all, this idea that the sadness does not have to be replaced by joy, but that both can be present simultaneously. And that these seemingly opposite emotions do not cancel each other out, but rather that each is a complement to the other, making the other even richer and more beautiful.

Loss is painful only because we loved, and I would not wish to erase the love in order to erase the pain. We are not free to choose all our circumstances - or to always save the ones we love - but we can choose to help others, to notice beauty, and to wrest hope from an often disappointing and fickle world.

Every day I think of what Cariana taught me – and what she is still teaching me. Thinking about all she went through in her short two-and-a-half years of life gives me inspiration to keep moving forward. She taught me the meaning of unconditional love, to accept others and myself in spite of our imperfections, and to find something of value in everyone I meet. She taught me the importance of reaching out and making connections with people around me, even though I had grown up feeling excluded and alone. She taught me that I can allow joy into my life, and even embrace it, without feeling that I have to leave the sadness behind. These are lessons that some people wait a lifetime to learn, and I will be forever grateful that Cariana chose to share her lifetime with me.

For anyone who is grieving now, it is important to know that it is possible to survive, to love, to laugh. We can be more than we think we can – more open in our hearts, more in tune with our true selves – and less limited by fears and by conformity. The only way to find what is out there waiting for you is to stay open. Live each day in a way that feels true to you, and look for the magic.

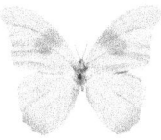

Epilogue

It has been fifteen years since Cariana was physically in my life, yet her presence is still as much a part of me as her absence. Grief still has an ebb and flow, as familiar as the underlying melancholy that has been present for most of my life: the haunting knowledge that in every moment there is some element of loss, something precious that will never come again in the exact same way. This feeling, which followed me even in childhood, became even stronger once I had children. They are now both in college, and I'm facing the poignancy of this lesson all over again as I watch them growing and thriving and moving a little bit farther away from me every day.

I will never stop missing Cariana. The "missing her" is always there, like music playing far away. Only the volume changes. Some days it is loud like a waterfall; other days it is more like a brook murmuring in the background. But even as I miss her, I also know that she is with me; in fact, that is probably the only thing in my life of which I am absolutely certain.

At first, I was confused about how I could go on, because I knew that I would never get over her death. Then I realized that I didn't have to get over it; I could simply carry her with me, not just as a memory but as an actual part of me. Everything I learned from her is incorporated in me, part of my body, as much a part of me as my own heartbeat.

Acknowledgments

This book would not exist without the three loves of my life: Placido, Liesl, and Cariana. I cannot thank them enough for all they have given me. Cariana inspired the book and gave me the strength to both write it and return to it, again and again, to hone and refine it. Placi and Liesl gave me the support I needed to keep trying, and the unconditional love that made me feel I could do it.

I am grateful to those who did not run away from my pain: Darlene, who met me for breakfast week in and week out for many years; and Cathy, who emailed me every Friday without fail since that terrible day, and continues to this day. And for all my friends — especially Jenny, Amy, and Maurice, who did not know Cariana personally, but whose expressions of love and caring, large and small, give me hope in what can be a discouraging world.

I am forever grateful for all the wonderful doctors, nurses, and therapists who cared for Cariana tenderly and never gave up hope.

I am grateful to the staff at Gerard's House, especially Katrina Koehler, who gave my children and I a place where we could express our pain without having to hide it.

I am grateful for my sister, Susan Scheppler, and all my extended family; and for my First Presbyterian church family, including the beloved Circle of Friends.

I am grateful for the Rev. Matt Davis who visited us in the hospital and for the Rev. Dr. Sheila Gustafson, whose courageous sermon at Cariana's funeral will forever be in my heart because she explained to everyone there how "this was not for the best."

I am grateful to the Rev. Dr. Harry Eberts for picking up that mantel and continuing to give that message. And I am grateful to the Rev. Linda Loving for encouraging and inspiring me as only a fellow writer and spiritual seeker can.

I am grateful to Karen Bomm for believing in me even though it was clear I did not have time to market a book.

I will always be grateful to Dave for creating these loving and amazing children with me.

And I am grateful to God for guiding me and walking with me even when I falter.

About the Author

Janis Gonzales is a mother, author, pediatrician, and public health physician with expertise in health policy, program management and administration. Her interests include children with special healthcare needs, prevention of adverse childhood events, and advocating for health equity and health in all policies. Janis currently works as the Maternal Child Health Director in the New Mexico Department of Health. She received her MD from the University of Illinois, her MPH from the University of New Mexico, and is Board Certified by the American Board of Pediatrics. She has been a Fellow of the American Academy of Pediatrics (AAP) for over 20 years, received the 2018 Early Childhood Champion Award from the AAP, and is the 2018-2020 President of the NM Pediatric Society (NM Chapter of the AAP). She lives in Santa Fe, NM with her children Placido and Liesl.

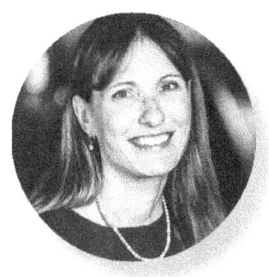 ...*more from Dr. Gonzales!*

This story of my daughter's life has become a springboard to discuss broad-ranging topics such as the practice of medicine, the power of prayer, the search for guidance, and the need for connection. This book is a deeply personal look at the depths of grief and the possibilities of hope.

If you relate to my story, I would love to hear from you. Here are a few ways you can reach out to me!

   www.facebook.com/janisgonzalesauthor

   twitter.com/janisgonzalesmd

   www.linkedin.com/in/janisgonzalesmd/

www.AGentleLife.com

www.ingramcontent.com/pod-product-compliance
Lightning Source LLC
Chambersburg PA
CBHW052059070526
44584CB00017B/2254